CONCEPTS OF MEDICAL-SURGICAL NURSING

The RN NCLEX Review Series

Brenda Goodner, R.N., M.S.N., C.S.

SKIDMORE-ROTH PUBLISHING, INC.

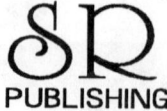
PUBLISHING

Cover design: Larissa Rodriguez

Copyright © 1994 by Skidmore-Roth Publishing, Inc. All rights reserved. No part of this book may be copied or transmitted in any form or by any means without written permission from the publisher.

Notice: The author and publisher of this volume have taken care to make certain that all information is correct and compatible with standards generally accepted at the time of publication.

Goodner, Brenda
The RN NCLEX Series: Medical-Surgical Nursing/Brenda Goodner

ISBN 0-944132-85-5
1. Nursing Handbooks, Manuals
2. Medical Handbooks, Manuals

SKIDMORE-ROTH PUBLISHING, INC.
7730 Trade Center Ave.
El Paso, Texas 79912
1 (800)825-3150

TABLE OF CONTENTS

UNIT 1
Respiratory System
Adult Respiratory Distress Syndrome (ARDS) 2
Bronchogenic Carcinoma (Lung Cancer) 6
Carbon Monoxide Poisoning 10
Chronic Obstructive Pulmonary Disease (COPD) 13
Pneumonia 22
Pneumothorax 26
Pulmonary Embolism 29
Respiratory Acidosis 34
Tracheostomy 37
Tuberculosis 43
General Study Questions 47

UNIT 2
Cardiovascular System
Angina Pectoris 60
Cardiac Failure
   • Left-Sided 64
   • Right-Sided 67
Congestive Heart Failure 70
Hypertension 74
Myocardial Infarction 77
Pulmonary Edema 83
General Study Questions 86

UNIT 3
Immune System
Acquired Immunodeficiency Syndrome (AIDS) 92
Anaphylaxis 97
Infection 101
Systemic Lupus Erythematosus (SLE) 105

UNIT 4
Hematologic System
Anemia 110
Disseminated Intravascular Coagulopathy (DIC) 113
Leukemia 117
Pernicious Anemia 122
Sickle Cell Anemia 126

UNIT 5
Nervous System
Alzheimer's Disease 134
Cerebrovascular Accident 139
Head Injury 146
Myasthenia Gravis 150
Parkinson's Disease 154

UNIT 6
Endocrine System
Diabetes Mellitus 160
Hypothyroidism 170
SIADH 174
General Study Questions 177

UNIT 7
Musculoskeletal System
Cast 188
Compartment Syndrome 192
Fractures 195
Osteoarthritis 200
Osteomyelitis 204
Traction 207

UNIT 8
Urinary/Renal System
Pyelonephritis 212
Renal Calculi 214
Renal Failure 217
Urinary Tract Infection 220
General Study Questions 224

UNIT 9
Gastrointestinal System
Peptic Ulcers 236
Cirrhosis of the Liver 241
Hepatitis A 245
Hepatitis B 248
General Study Questions 251

UNIT 10
Male & Female Reproductive Systems
Hysterectomy 260
Ovarian Cancer 263
Toxic Shock Syndrome 266
Prostatitis 269
Prostate Cancer 272
Benign Prostatic Hyperplasia (Hypertrophy) 275

UNIT 11
The Eye and Ear
Cataracts 280
Glaucoma 285
Meniere's Disease 290
Otitis Media 294
General Study Questions 295

UNIT 12
Concepts of Special Concern
Burns 304
Cancer 308
Hemorrhage 318
Hypovolemic Shock 323
Informed Consent 326
Lead Poisoning 329
Malignant Hyperthermia 332
Pain 335
Shock 344
Metabolic Alkalosis 349

UNIT 13
Comprehensive Test
General Test Questions to Prepare
the Student for the NCLEX 352

INDEX 417

INTRODUCTION TO NCLEX

- What to Know about NCLEX
- Study skills
- Six Stumbling Blocks to Test Taking and How to Avoid Them
- How to Use this Book

What to Know about the NCLEX

✦ All candidates will take the NCLEX on a computer.

✦ The test will involve a minimum of 75 correctly answered questions or a maximum of five hours for completion. Reportedly, when you have answered the correct number of questions, the computer will tell you that you have completed the test.

✦ All RN candidates in the United States take the same test.

✦ The questions are all multiple choice.

✦ Candidates must answer each question. It is not possible to proceed on to the next question without having answered the current one, and it is not possible to go back and answer a previous question.

✦ At this time, the passing score is 1600.

✦ You must retake the entire exam if a combined score of 1600 is not achieved on the first attempt.

✦ Each state determines how many times you may retake the test. Check with your state board for restrictions.

✦ The score will be reported to you only as a "pass" or "fail". The numerical score is not given. If you fail, your notice will be accompanied by a continuum which will show how you scored on each part of the nursing process: high, low, and pass.

✦ You will probably receive your test results in about 30 days.

✦ The Board of Nursing in the state where you write the exam will grant licensure.

✦ NCLEX stands for the National Council Licensure Examination.

The State Board MATRIX

The NCLEX questions are based on two major components of nursing knowledge:
- The Nursing Process
- Client Needs

The Nursing Process

The four phases of the nursing process are:

✦ **Assessment:** Collection of data, analysis of data, use of data to formulate and prioritize Nursing Diagnoses.

✦ **Outcome Criteria:** Measurable short and long-term goals are established.

✦ **Interventions:** Nursing actions to ensure the attainment of the established goals.

✦ **Evaluation:** Analysis of expected outcome as to successful completion. Revision of nursing care plan if needed.

The Nursing Process at a Glance

Assessment questions involve:
- Gathering data
- Listening to patient and family
- Observation
- Reading lab reports and chart

Planning questions involve:
- Analyzing data
- Setting short-term and long-term goals
- Recognizing abnormal data

Intervention questions involve:
- Nursing actions
- Independent nursing care

Evaluation questions involve:
- Patient's response to treatment
- Achievement of goals

Client Needs

There are four categories of basic health needs:

Safe, effective care environment. This category includes:
- Safety
- Preparation in treatments
- Safe procedures
- Quality assurance
- Goal-oriented care

Physiological integrity. This category includes:
- Physiological adaptation
- Comfort
- Mobility
- Providing basic care

Psychosocial integrity. This category includes:
- Psychosocial adaptation
- Comfort
- Mobility
- Providing basic care

Health promotion and maintenance. This category includes:
- Self-care
- Support systems
- Continued growth and development
- Prevention and early treatment of diseases

The NCLEX exam is constructed as follows:
- Safe, effective care environment: 25-31%
- Physiological integrity: 42-48%
- Psychosocial integrity: 9-15%
- Health promotion and maintenance: 12-18%

Level of Clinical Skill

Approximately 80% of the exam tests application of knowledge and analysis of data, including establishing of priorities. The other 20% is recall and comprehension. These review questions are constructed to reflect this testing pattern. The levels of cognitive and clinical skill utilized in developing these questions are:

1. Knowledge—Basic recall of information.
2. Comprehension—Basic understanding of information and relationships.
3. Application—Applying knowledge to patient care in specific situations.
4. Analysis and synthesis—Understanding rationale upon which decisions are based and putting the parts of data together.

Study Skills

1. Control your environment. Do whatever it takes to find a quiet place to study. Get up early in the morning, while everyone is asleep, or find a nook at the library.
2. Block a specific time for study. Study your biorhythms to know the time of day you are functioning at peak performance.
3. Become part of a small, dedicated study group; 3-5 people is optimal.
4. Tackle difficult concepts first, before you get tired.
5. Get enough sleep.
6. Eat right, especially protein, complex carbohydrates, and glucose ("brain food").
7. Avoid any medications or stimulants if possible.
8. Study key concepts by asking yourself, "What are four different ways this concept could be tested?"

9. Think NURSING PROCESS—Each question is based on the nursing process. Ask yourself "How could this concept be tested according to the nursing process?" or "What does a nurse need to know about this concept."

10. Study all of the information included in the rationale. Ask: "How could this information be tested?"

How to Take the Test

- Tell yourself you know more than you do.
- Take the question as it is; do not assume information that is not there.
- Note key words in the stem; analyze what the question is asking.
- While choosing the correct answer, rationalize why the other detractors are wrong.
- Go with your first impression or hunch if you are not sure.
- Guess if you do not know.
- Practice relaxation techniques throughout the test.
- If you feel panicky after confronting two or three questions you do not know, take a few deep, diaphragmatic breaths before starting again.
- Keep telling yourself, "I know more than I think I know."

SIX STUMBLING BLOCKS TO TEST TAKING
...and how to avoid them!

- **Answering the question too quickly without analyzing the distractors**

    If you find you are overlooking details, or misreading the question or key concepts, you may be reading the question too quickly and jumping to conclusions. You need to slow down and double check everything.

- **Failing to read all of the distractors**

    Look at each wrong distractor carefully. Examine it and determine why it cannot be the right answer.

- **Giving up too soon; failing to reason out the answer if you think you don't know it**

    Do you lack the information or the data base? Do not panic. Make a reasonable guess. Often, you can rule out wrong distractors.

- **Failing to analyze key words**

    Ask yourself, "What is the most important phrase in this question?"

- **Inferring data that is not present in the question**

    If you inferred data that was not presented in the question or made assumptions about the patient situation, you were "reading into" the question. If you normally make this type of error, you should select the answer carefully. Computerized testing will not allow you to go back and change answers.

❐ Identifying priorities in the wrong order

Identifying priorities in the wrong order may cause confusion over minor points that may just be thrown into a patient situation. Ask: "Which of these priorities will result in injury or death if not addressed?" Remember the ABC's. Ask yourself: "Which intervention is a priority in the well-being of the patient?"

HOW TO USE THIS BOOK

This book was written on the concept format, addressing the concepts in medical-surgical nursing that tend to be frequently tested on the National Council Licensure Examination (NCLEX). Emphasis is placed on nursing assessments and interventions because an estimated 65% of the questions on state boards are drawn from these two parts of the nursing process.

In studying each concept, ask yourself, "How could this information be tested?" or "What are three or four different ways this information can be tested?" For example, in the patient with ARDS, review the assessment and make up questions on how dyspnea, breath sounds, and level of consciousness can be tested. Apply the same technique with the information given in the stem and rationale of each question.

The questions presented were written not just to give you the answer but to give information in the question and rationale that can help you in answering any question regarding the concept.

ACKNOWLEDGEMENTS

I would like to express special gratitude to three individuals who were instrumental in the production of this book. Loretta Diehl, RN, MSN, of New Mexico State University at Alamogordo, reviewed the manuscript with meticulous attention and expertise, adding important content throughout. My editorial assistant, Alexandra Swann, was invaluable in the production of the book: researching information, pulling the questions and concepts together, and handling the final production details. Larissa Rodriguez created the style for the book and her typesetting assistance gave organization to the information presented. Their invaluable assistance made this project a pleasure to produce.

Brenda Goodner

UNIT 1
RESPIRATORY SYSTEM

- Adult Respiratory Distress Syndrome (ARDS)
- Bronchogenic Carcinoma
- Carbon Monoxide Poisoning
- Chronic Obstructive Pulmonary Disease (COPD)
- Pneumonia
- Pneumothorax
- Pulmonary Embolism
- Respiratory Acidosis
- Tracheostomy
- Tuberculosis

ADULT RESPIRATORY DISTRESS SYNDROME

DEFINITION
A syndrome of altered respiratory function characterized by:
- Reduced perfusion
- Increased capillary permeability
- Direct tissue and capillary injury
- Loss of compliance with widespread atelectasis

PATHOPHYSIOLOGY
Pulmonary injury leads to increased capillary congestion, permeability, and edema and affects surfactant-producing cells. Stiffening of the lungs, atelectasis and edema occur, producing the profound hypoxemia of this syndrome.

ASSOCIATED MEDICAL CONDITIONS
- Sepsis
- Pneumonia
- Smoke inhalation
- Increasing intracranial pressure
- Trauma
- Shock
- Fat embolus
- Anaphylaxis
- Pregnancy-induced hypertension
- Poisoning

ASSESSMENT
- Increasing respiratory rate (early sign)
- Hypoxemia (even with High O_2 administration)
- ABGs: Especially, gradual drop in PaO_2 and increase in $PaCO_2$
- Severe dyspnea
- Cyanosis
- Changes in level of consciousness
- Adventitious breath sounds:
  - Inspiratory crackles (early stage)
  - Widespread crackles (late stage)
  - Bilateral infiltrates

CLIENT NEED
Physiological integrity

NURSING INTERVENTIONS
- Monitor for life-threatening changes
- Provide chest physiotherapy
- Place in semi or high Fowler's to maximize thoracic excursion
- Provide supportive therapy for anxiety and fear
- Encourage rest to minimize O_2 consumption
- If on PEEP:
  - Monitor constantly
  - Administer medication (Morphine, Ativan, Diprivan and Pavulon) to decrease resistance to PEEP
  - Anticipate need for pain medication
  - Anticipate need for comfort, positioning needs
- Monitor mechanical ventilation (PEEP)
- Administer O_2 at high flow, 8-10 L/min (often with ventilator ET PEEP)
- Suction prn
- Encourage fluid intake (may be balanced with diuretics due to pulmonary edema)
- Meticulous eye care (Pavulon inhibits blink reflex) to decrease risk of corneal abrasions
- Monitor pulmonary artery pressure monitoring

PATIENT TEACHING
- Methods of communication
- Explanation of all procedures and equipment being implemented
- Drug therapy
- Conditions that might contribute to development of ARDS

ASSOCIATED NURSING DIAGNOSES

- Activity intolerance
- Hopelessness
- Anxiety, R/T ARDS, intubation and discomfort from PEEP
- Coping, ineffective individual
- Cardiac output, decreased R/T decreased venous return
- Dysfunctional ventilatory weaning response
- Ventilation, inability to sustain spontaneous
- Tissue perfusion, altered, cardiopulmonary
- Nutrition, altered: less than body requirements, R/T increased need and effect of intubation on caloric intake
- Fear
- Powerlessness
- Communication, impaired verbal, R/T airway management
- Gas exchange, impaired, R/T ARDS
- Self-care deficit: bathing/hygiene, dressing/grooming, feeding, toileting
- Breathing pattern, ineffective, R/T altered lung/thoracic pressure relationship
- Spiritual distress (distress of the human spirit)
- Sensory/perceptual alterations (olfactory)

STUDY QUESTIONS

■ Which electrolyte imbalance is the ARDs patient most likely to experience?
1. Metabolic acidosis
2. Metabolic alkalosis
3. Respiratory acidosis
4. Respiratory alkalosis

Answer: 4. Respiratory alkalosis

Rationale: The ARDs patient experiences tachypnea and hyperventilation, which results in excessive blowing off of CO_2, leading to respiratory alkalosis.

Nursing process: Evaluation

Client need: Physiological integrity

Clinical skill level: 3

■ The nurse assesses a gradual decrease in PaO_2 in the ARDS patient despite the administration of O_2 at 10L/min. This assessment indicates a potential complication because:
   1. O_2 level is too high
   2. Breathing is not spontaneous
   3. O_2 administration should be higher
   4. Response to O_2 is not positive

Answer: 4. Response to O_2 is not positive

Rationale: When PaO_2 does not go up with administration of high flow O_2, it indicates the oxygen is not being perfused in the body and a potential threat exists.

Nursing process: Evaluation

Client need: Physiological integrity

Clinical skill level: 4

■ The care plan instructs the nurse to monitor a patient suffering ARDS following massive body trauma. The first signs of ARDS are:
   1. Tachypnea and restlessness
   2. Cyanosis and diaphoresis
   3. Agitation and anger
   4. Confusion and seizures

Answer: 1. Tachypnea and restlessness

Rationale: Tachypnea and restlessness may indicate the early stage of hypoxia and the onset of ARDS. Early intervention can prevent later complications that dyspnea, cyanosis and diaphoresis often signal.

Client need: Physiological integrity

Nursing process: Assessment

Clinical skill level: 3

BRONCHOGENIC CARCINOMA (LUNG CANCER)

DEFINITION
Bronchogenic carcinoma is a malignancy of the lungs. Cancer of the larger bronchi is associated with cigarette smoking while cancer of the peripheral bronchi occurs almost equally in nonsmokers as smokers.

PATHOPHYSIOLOGY
Lung cancer is classified by cell type: (1) squamous cell carcinoma (2) oat cell carcinoma (3) adenocarcinoma (4) undifferentiated carcinoma. The treatment and prognosis depends upon the cell type. Prognosis is better with squamous cell (or epidermal) and adenocarcinoma than with the undifferentiated tumors.

ASSOCIATED MEDICAL CONDITIONS
- Asbestosis
- Emphysema

ASSESSMENT
- Cough (most common symptom):
  - Early disease: hacking, nonproductive
  - Late disease: thick, purulent sputum
  - Blood-tinged sputum (from the ulcerated tumor)
- Wheezing (from tumor obstructing bronchi)
- Repeated respiratory tract infections
- Fever (caused by infection)
- Hoarseness (laryngeal nerve involvement)
- Tightness in chest
- Hypoxia
- Dysphagia
- Edema around neck
- Chest pain (a late sign and related to bone metastasis)
- Pleural vision

Late signs:
- Weakness
- Anorexia
- Weight loss
- Anemia

CLIENT NEED
Physiological integrity

NURSING INTERVENTIONS
- Airway management
- Chest-tube management
- Pain management
- Provide O₂ or aerosol therapy
- Encourage deep breathing, coughing
- Protection from infection
- Nutritional support

MEDICAL INTERVENTIONS
- Bronchoscopy
- Chemotherapy
- Surgery: Lobectomy or pneumonectomy
- CT scan
- Radiation therapy

PATIENT TEACHING
- Persons who smoke or who work around asbestos should have chest x-rays once a year
- Preoperative teaching
- Risk of smoking
- Early detection and screening

ASSOCIATED NURSING DIAGNOSES
- Activity intolerance
- Denial, ineffective
- Gas exchange, impaired
- Fatigue
- Infection, high risk for
- Powerlessness
- Spiritual distress (distress of the human spirit)
- Anxiety
- Hopelessness
- Breathing pattern, ineffective
- Fear
- Pain, chronic
- Social isolation
- Tissue perfusion, altered, cardiopulmonary

■ Hoarseness is a sign of cancer. When it occurs in a patient with lung cancer, it is indicative of:
1. Metastatic pressure on the laryngeal nerve
2. Oat cell carcinoma with complications
3. Destruction of vocal cords by radiation
4. Side effects of radiation treatment

Answer: 1. Metastatic pressure on the laryngeal nerve

Rationale: Metastasis to the mediastinal lymph nodes causes nerve compression and eventually will cause vocal paralysis.

Client need: Physiological integrity

Nursing process: Evaluation

Clinical skill level: 4

■ The patient has been recently diagnosed with lung cancer, and the nurse checks the classification on the chart. Which histologic types of lung cancer have the poorest prognosis?
1. Squamous cell
2. Oat cell
3. Adenocarcinoma
4. Large cell

Answer: 2. Oat cell

Rationale: Oat cell, or small cell, metastasizes very quickly and very widely. It spreads to lymph nodes, bone marrow, liver and CNS, often before diagnosis is made.

Nursing process: Assessment

Client need: Physiological integrity

Clinical skill level: 2

■ The patient who has smoked 2 packs/day for 22 years states he has a "cigarette cough" that has worsened over the last 2-3 months and is now a productive cough. This complaint alerts the nurse to which sign of lung cancer?
   1. A cough that changes
   2. A dry cough
   3. A persistent cough
   4. A cough that causes hoarseness

Answer: 1. A cough that changes

Rationale: The "cigarette cough" begins as a dry, hacking, non-productive cough. When cancer develops, the cough becomes thick, purulent, blood-tinged.

Nursing process: Evaluation

Client need: Physiological integrity

Clinical skill level: 2

■ A recently-diagnosed patient has been told by the physician that lung cancer has metastasized to the lymph nodes and bone marrow. Radiation has been ordered. The major reason for treatment at this point is:
   1. Experimental
   2. Curative
   3. Palliative
   4. Unethical

Answer: 3. Palliative

Rationale: Radiation or chemotherapy is prescribed to reduce the tumor, thereby decreasing pain and pressure on vital structures affected by the metastasis.

Nursing process: Evaluation

Client need: Physiological integrity

Clinical skill level: 3

CARBON MONOXIDE POISONING

DEFINITION
Alteration in tissue perfusion and hypoxia as a result of inhalation of toxic levels of carbon monoxide gas from exhaust of cars or faulty gas heaters in a non-ventilated environment.

PATHOPHYSIOLOGY
The affinity of carbon monoxide for hemoglobin is 200 times that of oxygen. The displacement of oxygen by carbon monoxide leads to decreased uptake and delivery of oxygen, and hypoxemia occurs at the tissue level.

ASSESSMENT
- Headaches
- Syncope
- Convulsions
- Thermoregulation abnormalities
- Confusion
- Coma
- Cherry-red skin (early sign)
- Tachycardia and hypotension

CLIENT NEED
Physiological integrity

NURSING INTERVENTIONS
- Administer O_2 100%
- Provide rest to decrease O_2 demand
- Neurological assessments for signs and symptoms of increasing intracranial pressure
- Prepare for ventilator
- Seizure precautions

MEDICAL INTERVENTIONS
- Carboxyhemoglobin levels drawn
- Ventilator management
- Cardiovascular monitoring

PATIENT TEACHING
- Importance of follow-up
- Evaluation of home environment for presence of carbon monoxide levels

ASSOCIATED NURSING DIAGNOSES
- Anxiety
- Poisoning, high risk for
- Trauma, high risk for
- Tissue perfusion, altered (cerebral, cardiopulmonary)
- Fear
- Suffocation, high risk for
- Cardiac output, decreased

STUDY QUESTIONS

■ Carbon monoxide causes tissue hypoxia. Poisoning occurs when the carbon monoxide:
1. Cannot carry oxygen to the blood
2. Overwhelms O_2 transport
3. Saps hemoglobin from the cells
4. Molecules are larger than O_2 molecules

Answer: 2. Overwhelms O_2 transport

Rationale: Carbon monoxide has a strong affinity for hemoglobin and binds to it. This prevents O_2-CO_2 exchange, and the cells become hypoxic and die.

Nursing process: Assessment

Client need: Physiological integrity

Clinical skill level: 2

■ The priority of care in the person experiencing carbon monoxide poisoning is administration of:
1. Oxygen
2. Narcan
3. Normal saline
4. Lactated Ringer's

Answer: 1. Oxygen

Rationale: Oxygen is the antidote for carbon monoxide poisoning and should be administered in high concentrations.

Client need: Physiological integrity

Nursing process: Intervention

Clinical skill level: 3

CHRONIC OBSTRUCTIVE PULMONARY DISEASE (COPD)

DEFINITION
COPD is a progressively debilitating disease that is incurable. The diagnosis includes three different disorders: Emphysema, asthma, and chronic bronchitis.

PATHOPHYSIOLOGY
Asthma: Characterized by bronchoconstriction that is reversible with medication. During exacerbations, the patient experiences wheezing, coughing, and dyspnea. A variety of chemical (including histamine) meditors cause bronchial constriction and a reversible inflammatory response.

Chronic bronchitis: Characterized by a productive cough that lasts for at least 2 years. Bacterial infections reoccur. Recurrent infections cause secretions and, eventually, obstruction. Atelectasis and fibrosis (from scarring of lung tissue) results and hypoxemia occurs.

Emphysema: Characterized by permanent hyperinfection and destruction of alveoli; eventually resulting in impaired diffusion of oxygen and inadequate O_2-CO_2 exchange. Hyperinflation causes the rupture of alveoli and collapses the capillary bed where O_2-CO_2 exchange occurs. Coughing is inadequate to remove secretions and chronic infections result. Complications include right-sided heart failure (cor pulmonale).

MOST COMMON MEDICAL CONDITIONS
- Emphysema
- Chronic bronchitis
- Asthma

ASSESSMENT

- Dyspnea on exertion
- Pulse rate
- Neck vein engorgement
- Productive cough (color, consistency)
- Wheezing
- Weight loss
- Pain
- Respiratory rate
- Fatigue
- Peripheral edema
- Cyanosis (face, nails, earlobes)
- Tachypnea
- Dependent edema

CLIENT NEED

Physiological integrity

NURSING INTERVENTIONS

- Force fluids
- Postural drainage
- Encourage pursed-lip and diaphragmatic breathing
- Administer O_2 cautiously (especially in emphysema when stimulus to breathe is reversed)
- Administer antibiotics
- Administer IPPB if ordered
- Encourage intermittent periods of rest and activity

PATIENT TEACHING

- Avoid smoking cigarettes
- Get flu shots every year
- Explain reason for prophylactic antibiotics (if prescribed)
- Wear mask if in a polluted environment
- Avoid people who are prone to infections
- Increase in dyspnea
- Teach purpose of diaphragmatic and pursed-lip breathing
- Teach early symptoms to report to physician:
    - Change in sputum production
    - Tightness in chest
    - Chest pain
    - Increasing fatigue

ASSOCIATED NURSING DIAGNOSES

- Activity intolerance
- Fatigue
- Aspiration, high risk for
- Hopelessness
- Powerlessness
- Nutrition: less than body requirements, altered
- Ventilation, inability to sustain spontaneous
- Anxiety
- Fear
- Gas exchange, impaired
- Infection, high risk for
- Physical mobility, impaired
- Tissue perfusion, altered: cardiopulmonary, peripheral

STUDY QUESTIONS

Aminophylline is prescribed to the patient with respiratory problems. This medication acts as a:

1. Pain reliever
2. Bronchodilator
3. Broncho constrictor
4. Cough suppressant

Answer: 2. Bronchodilator

Rationale: Aminophylline (theophylline) acts by relaxing the smooth muscle in the bronchial airways and blood vessels throughout the pulmonary system.

Nursing process: Intervention

Client need: Physiological integrity

Clinical skill level: 2

- The patient with COPD responds to hypoxia by developing which possible complication?
  1. Hypotension
  2. Enlarged liver
  3. Enlarged left ventricle
  4. Polycythemia

  Answer: 4. Polycythemia

  Rationale: Hypoxemia caused by COPD stimulates the production of red blood cells, and polycythemia develops. Polycythemia is the accumulation of too many red blood cells in the body. Phlebotomy is the initial treatment, sometimes followed by chemotherapy to produce myelosuppression.

  Nursing process: Intervention

  Client need: Physiological integrity

  Clinical skill level: 2

- COPD causes hypertrophy of the heart. Which chamber is most likely affected?
  1. AV chamber
  2. SA chamber
  3. Right ventricle
  4. Left ventricle

  Answer: 3. Right ventricle

  Rationale: Vasoconstriction in the pulmonary vessels occurs due to decreased PaO_2. This, in turn, results in pulmonary hypertension. The right ventricle must keep increasing pressure to eject blood into the constricted pulmonary vessels. Eventually, the increasing pressure results in right ventricle failure.

  Nursing process: Assessment

  Client need: Physiological integrity

  Clinical skill level: 2

■ The nurse instructs the person with chronic obstructive pulmonary disease (COPD) to breathe:
1. At an increased rate within comfortable limits
2. With an open mouth during inspiration
3. While pursing lips during expiration
4. With an increased time of inspiration

Answer: 3. While pursing lips during expiration

Rationale: Pursed-lip breathing allows for longer expiration and more time for O_2-CO_2 exchange.

Nursing process: Intervention

Client need: Physiological integrity

Clinical skill level: 2

■ An initial nursing assessment of the COPD patient reveals a potential complication. It is:
1. He has never smoked cigarettes
2. His hemoglobin is 16 g/100 ml
3. His respiratory rate is 20 breaths/minute
4. His wife smokes two packs of cigarettes a day

Answer: 4. His wife smokes two packs of cigarettes a day

Rationale: Secondary smoke is believed to be almost as harmful as actually inhaling the smoke.

Nursing process: Evaluation

Client need: Physiological integrity

Clinical skill level: 2

■ A patient has chronic obstructive pulmonary disease (COPD). He constantly complains of coughing, fatigue, and sputum production. During the assessment, the nurse observes his breathing pattern. She notes the barrel-chest that is common in COPD patients. Which evaluation would best explain these signs and symptoms?
1. Ruptured bleb of the lung
2. Presence of an infection in the lung
3. An acute attack of asthma
4. Excessive residual volume of trapped air in the lung

Answer: 4. Excessive residual volume of trapped air in the lung

Rationale: In COPD air is trapped in the alveoli, and the patient uses accessory muscles to attempt to exhale the trapped air. This causes an increased diameter of the thorax, resulting in barrel chest.

Nursing process: Evaluation

Client need: Physiological integrity

| Clinical skill level: 2 |

■ A patient suffering asthma has been prescribed theophylline. In performing a general health assessment, which factor will be of most importance?
1. The patient is age 18
2. The patient is female
3. The patient is obese
4. The patient smokes

Answer: 4. The patient smokes

Rationale: Smoking reduces the effects of theophylline and a higher dose may be required for optimal effectiveness.

Nursing process: Assessment

Client need: Physiological integrity

| Clinical skill level: 3 |

■ The nurse teaches that the most common side effects of aminophylline therapy are:
1. Prolonged Q-T interval
2. Tachycardia, palpitation
3. Dry mouth, constipation
4. Hyperventilation, hyperkalemia

Answer: 2. Tachycardia, palpitation

Rationale: Being a sympathomimetic bronchodilator, aminophylline may cause tachycardia, palpitations, dysrhythmias, and hypertension.

Nursing process: Intervention

Client need: Physiological integrity

> Clinical skill level: 4

■ A patient is diagnosed with emphysema. The nurse is doing initial rounds and finds the patient is flushed, experiencing bradypnea and dyspnea. She notes the O_2 rate is 4L/min. Her first action is:
1. Call for help
2. Notify doctor stat
3. Turn O_2 to 2L/min
4. Get a BP reading

Answer: 3. Turn O_2 to 2L/min

Rationale: The patient suffering emphysema should be maintained on a low O_2 setting. In emphysema the breathing mechanism is reversed, and O_2 becomes the stimulus for breathing. If the patient is getting too much O_2 the stimulus disappears, dyspnea sets in, and breathing may stop.

Nursing process: Intervention

Client need: Physiological integrity

> Clinical skill level: 2

■ Which breath sounds does the nurse hear in a patient diagnosed with emphysema?
1. Rhonchi and expiratory wheezing
2. Crackles and expiratory wheezing
3. Rhonchi and inspiratory wheezing
4. No sounds related to alveoli destruction

Answer: 1. Rhonchi and expiratory wheezing

Rationale: Rhonchi are low-pitched sounds that are heard when air is forced through airways that are blocked by secretions.

Nursing process: Assessment

Client need: Physiological integrity

Clinical skill level: 2

■ In teaching an emphysema patient about his disease, the nurse is aware that certain changes in the lungs are characteristic of emphysema. The pathophysiology involves alveolar sacs that:
1. Collapse
2. Are fibrotic
3. Are filled with fluid
4. Are filled with CO_2

Answer: 1. Collapse

Rationale: Repeated infections that result from retained secretions and congestion causes either destruction or bloating of the alveoli. This increases pulmonary resistance and the airways collapse.

Nursing process: Evaluation

Client need: Physiological integrity

Clinical skill level: 2

■ The nurse assesses crackles throughout both lung fields. What treatment does the nurse initiate for this atelectasis?
1. Start 4 liters O_2
2. Initiate chest physiotherapy
3. Call physician for diuretics
4. Call physician for antibiotics

Answer: 2. Initiate chest physiotherapy

Rationale: Coughing, deep breathing, and postural drainage, which are all components of chest physiotherapy can open the alveoli and resolve the atelectasis, which is causing the abnormal lung sounds.

Nursing process: Intervention

Client need: Physiological integrity

Clinical skill level: 3

PNEUMONIA

DEFINITION
The inflammation and consolidation of lung tissue secondary to virus, bacteria, chemicals, food, fluids, or vomitus invading or entering the lungs.

PATHOPHYSIOLOGY
Microorganisms invade the lungs and become entrapped in the bronchi, then spread to the alveoli and through the lobe. Inhalation of organisms and aspiration of foreign materials are the most common causes of pneumonia. Consolidation is caused by exudate filling the alveolar spaces and leads to shunting of blood and hypoxemia.

ASSOCIATED MEDICAL CONDITIONS
- Bronchopneumonia
- Influenza
- Alcoholism
- Staphylococcal pneumonia (frequently nosocomial)
- Pneumococcal lobar pneumonia
- Leukemia
- Tracheostomy
- Aspiration pneumonia
- Pneumocystis carinii pneumonia (in AIDS patients)

ASSESSMENT
- Slight elevation in temperature (at onset)
- Increasing pulse
- Cyanosis
- Productive cough
- Fremitus
- Chills
- Changes in level of consciousness
- High fever (especially with bacterial pneumonia)
- Increasing respirations
- Nasal flaring
- Crackles (lower lungs)
- Blood-tinged sputum
- Profuse perspiration
- Intact gag reflex (especially before giving food or fluids)

CLIENT NEED
Physiological integrity

NURSING INTERVENTIONS
- Early ambulation
- Encourage use of incentive spirometer
- Provide oral hygiene
- Maintenance of oxygen therapy
- Monitor sputum analysis
- Monitor ABGs
- Monitor chest x-ray
- Administer antibiotics or penicillin (for pneumococcal)
- Good handwashing
- Postural drainage via percussion and vibration
- Implement use of humidifier
- High level of fluid intake encouraged
- Monitor temperature and sputum
- Administer oxygen therapy
- Ventilator management

PATIENT TEACHING
- Encourage influenza vaccine
- Quit smoking
- Importance of turning, coughing and deep breathing
- Importance of keeping appointment for check-ups
- How to cough effectively
- Avoid excessive alcohol intake
- Nutrition
- Avoiding exposure (i.e. crowds, children if immunocompromised)
- Importance of taking medication exactly as prescribed
- Get refills when needed

ASSOCIATED NURSING DIAGNOSES
- Anxiety
- Body temperature, high risk for altered
- Infection, high risk for
- Pain
- Tissue perfusion, altered (cardiopulmonary)
- Fatigue
- Nutrition: less than body requirements, altered
- Knowledge deficit
- Ineffective airway clearance

STUDY QUESTIONS

■ Pneumonia is a frequent complication when a patient is immobilized. Which cardinal sign is indicative of this condition?
1. Dyspnea
2. Hypothermia
3. Hypertension
4. Hypotension

Answer: 1. Dyspnea

Rationale: Although difficulty in breathing is common to respiratory disorders, it is always an early sign of pneumonia.

Nursing process: Assessment

Client need: Physiological integrity

Clinical skill level: 2

■ Crackles are abnormal lung sounds that will be heard in a patient with:
1. Asthma
2. Friction rub
3. Pneumonia
4. Tactile fremitus

Answer: 3. Pneumonia

Rationale: Crackles indicate there is fluid in the lungs, usually more obvious on inspiration and in pneumonia, heard at the base of the lungs.

Nursing process: Assessment

Client need: Physiological integrity

Clinical skill level: 3

- Pneumonia is the result of a bacterial infection when the nurse assesses the sputum to be:
    1. Thin, white, and frothy
    2. Thick, black, and viscous
    3. Thin, rusty, and frothy
    4. Thick, yellow, and frothy

    Answer: 3. Thin, rusty, and frothy

    Rationale: Pneumococcal pneumonia produces a rusty brown or blood streaked sputum.

    Nursing process: Evaluation

    Client need: Physiological integrity

    Clinical skill level: 3

PNEUMOTHORAX

DEFINITION
The escape of air from a lung into the pleural cavity. This condition usually results from an injury to the lung, and the seriousness of the condition depends upon the extent of thoracic injury.

PATHOPHYSIOLOGY
The various types of pneumothoraces often result from fractured ribs which damage internal organs or as a result of spontaneous rupture of pulmonary blebs.

ASSOCIATED MEDICAL CONDITIONS
- Hemothorax
- Tension pneumothorax
- Emphysema
- Hemopneumothorax
- Open pneumothorax
- Iatrogenic secondary to subclavian central line insertion

ASSESSMENT
- Shortness of breath
- Anxiety
- Tachycardia
- Chest pain
- Breath sounds absent, distant
- Deviation of larynx, trachea away from point of injury
- History of recent trauma
- Tachypnea
- Chest tightness
- Restlessness
- Cyanosis
- Tympanitic percussion on affected side
- Chest asymmetric (affected side restricted and somewhat bloated in appearance)

CLIENT NEED
Physiological integrity

NURSING INTERVENTIONS

- Monitor wound carefully
- Pain management
- Administer antibiotics as per physician's orders and monitor
- Assist in thoracentesis
- Prepare for auto blood transfusion
- Maintenance of oxygen therapy
- Chest-tube management
- Assist in chest tube placement (in the fourth through sixth intercostal space)
- Prepare for thoracotomy

PATIENT TEACHING

- Inform patient of acceptable activities
- Eliminate behaviors which may have led to fractures and trauma; i.e. drug abuse; DWI

ASSOCIATED NURSING DIAGNOSES

- Anxiety
- Fear
- Gas exchange, impaired
- Hypoxia R/T diminished surface area for gas exchange
- Injury, high risk for
- Airway clearance, ineffective, R/T pain and guarding of chest movement
- Infection: at risk for R/T pulmonary trauma
- Cardiac output, decreased
- Pain
- Powerlessness
- Pain R/T chest tube and/or associated blunt trauma and rib fractures
- Breathing pattern, ineffective
- Nutrition: less than body requirements, R/T increased caloric needs for healing
- Tissue perfusion, cerebral, cardiopulmonary

STUDY QUESTIONS

- A patient comes to the ER complaining of difficulty breathing and chest pain. The patient denies any history of trauma. The nurse notes tracheal displacement. She immediately suspects:
    1. Flail chest
    2. Tension pneumothorax
    3. Myocardial infarction
    4. Status asthmaticus

    Answer: 2. Tension pneumothorax
    Rationale: The cardinal sign of tension pneumothorax is the displaced trachea. Tension pneumothorax is often caused by the rupture of an emphysematous bleb and can occur without trauma.
    Nursing process: Assessment
    Client need: Physiological integrity

    Clinical skill level: 3

- On initial rounds, the nurse notes the patient who has sustained an open pneumothorax from a stab wound experiencing dyspnea. Breath sounds reveal a high-pitched, crowing sound that she evaluates as inspiratory laryngeal stridor. Her next priority is:
    1. Call a code
    2. Notify the physician
    3. Turn up oxygen flow
    4. Check wound for hemorrhage

    Answer: 2. Notify the physician
    Rationale: Stridor is caused by laryngeal muscle spasms that can be obstructing the airway, causing an emergency that might require a tracheostomy and insertion of ET tube.
    Client need: Physiological integrity
    Nursing process: Intervention

    Clinical skill level: 4

PULMONARY EMBOLISM

DEFINITION
An embolism is a blood clot, a piece of fat, or particle of debris that breaks away from its original site and travels through the bloodstream, picking up particles and subsequently lodging in a vessel lumen causing obstruction of blood flow through the heart and/or to lung tissue.

PATHOPHYSIOLOGY
After traveling through the bloodstream, the embolus will pick up fat particles and other debris until it eventually becomes large enough that it gets stuck in the pulmonary artery. A respiratory emergency exists at this point.

ASSOCIATED MEDICAL CONDITIONS
- Fat embolism
- Multi-trauma
- Peripheral vascular disease
- Abdominal surgery, post-op
- Immobility
- Hypercoagulability

ASSESSMENT
- Dyspnea
- Stabbing chest pain
- Cyanosis
- Rapid, irregular pulse
- Dilates pupils
- Restlessness (a cardinal initial sign)
- Apprehension
- Diaphoresis
- Fear
- Dysrhythmias
- Hypoxia

CLIENT NEED
Physiological integrity

NURSING INTERVENTIONS

- Administer O₂ stat as this is a respiratory emergency
- Early ambulation (post-surgery) is the best prevention
- Closely monitor obese patients
- Do not massage legs; especially calf
- Pain management
- Maintenance/monitoring of anticoagulant therapy
- Establish IV line for administration of emergency medication
- Active/passive ROM, as indicated-antiembolic stockings (PAS)
- Closely monitor for signs of restlessness
- Maintain HOB elevation to promote ventilation
- Assess for Homan's sign
- Administer infusion Heparin sodium until partial thromboplastin time is 2 to 2.5 normal value (Coumadin for 3 to 6 months)

PATIENT TEACHING

- Do not take aspirin while on Coumadin
- Avoid restrictive clothing on legs and prolonged sitting or standing
- Teach signs of bleeding related to Coumadin intake
- Avoid smoking
- Use soft toothbrush, electric razor
- Avoid being bruised, constipated or engaging in behaviors that are potentially injurious i.e. contact sports
- Evaluation of contraceptive use in women of childbearing age

ASSOCIATED NURSING DIAGNOSES

- Activity intolerance
- Pain
- Powerlessness
- Tissue perfusion, altered (cardiopulmonary)
- Cardiac output, decreased
- Anxiety
- Fear
- Post-trauma response
- Ventilation, inacardiac output, decreasedbility to sustain spontaneous

STUDY QUESTIONS

■ Upon auscultation of the lungs, the nurse assesses a sound described as a "grating, not decreased or increased after coughing." This adventitious sound is:
1. Friction rub
2. Crackling
3. Rhonchi
4. Wheezing

Answer: 1. Friction rub
Rationale: This abnormal sound is often heard in conditions such as pleurisy and pulmonary embolism. Pleural friction rub has often been described as the sound heard when rubbing leather together.
Nursing process: Assessment
Client need: Physiological integrity

Clinical skill level: 3

■ The patient 2 days post-op from abdominal surgery is showing signs of anxiety and increased pain. The nurse is concerned because the patient is obese and has difficulty ambulating. A priority assessment is for:
1. Restlessness
2. Vomiting
3. Noncompliance
4. Increasing pain

Answer: 1. Restlessness
Rationale: Restlessness, probably related to early hypoxia, is the first cardinal indication of pulmonary embolism. Emergency treatment is still possible at this point.
Client need: Physiological integrity
Nursing process: Assessment

Clinical skill level: 4

■ What is the priority nursing intervention once the nurse assesses the patient is throwing a pulmonary embolus?
1. Administer 100% O₂
2. Prepare for chest tubes
3. Prepare for tracheostomy
4. Start IV for medications

Answer: 1. Administer 100% O₂

Rationale: This is a respiratory emergency and oxygen should be administered at a high flow rate.

Client need: Physiological integrity

Nursing process: Intervention

Clinical skill level: 3

■ The patient is being discharged on Coumadin therapy. The nurse instructs the patient to:
1. Keep the Protamine Sulfate antidote handy
2. Use in conjunction with Tylenol and/or Advil
3. Discontinue if bruises appear
4. Take the medicine at the same time each day

Answer: 4. Take the medicine at the same time each day

Rationale: Coumadin therapy affects the prothrombin time (PT) and if not taken at the same time every day, the anticoagulant effects may be altered. The PT should be 1.5-2 times normal.

Nursing process: Intervention

Client need: Physiological integrity

Clinical skill level: 3

■ Which nursing interventions are essential to prevent thrombus formation when caring for the patient with a problem of immobility?
1. Turn, cough, and deep breathe every 2 hours
2. Move the patient to a chair every 4 to 6 hours
3. Frequent passive and active range of motion
4. Place a pillow under the knees of the patient

Answer: 3. Frequent passive and active range of motion

Rationale: Circulation is the key to preventing the formation of a blood clot.

Nursing process: Intervention

Client need: Physiological integrity

Clinical skill level: 2

RESPIRATORY ACIDOSIS

DEFINITION
Respiratory acidosis is an acid-base imbalance resulting from any condition that causes hypoventilation. The pH is less than 7.35 mg while the $PaCO_2$ is greater than 45 mm Hg.

PATHOPHYSIOLOGY
Insufficient excretion of carbon dioxide and elevation cause high plasma carbon dioxide levels and increased carbonic acid levels. Chronic respiratory acidosis is often caused by chronic obstructive pulmonary disease (COPD) and may result from excessive amounts of oxygen given to COPD patients. Excessive production of CO_2 resulting from a high metabolic rate or high production of carbohydrate may also lead to respiratory acidosis.

MOST COMMON MEDICAL CONDITIONS
- COPD
- Hypermetabolism
- Airway obstruction
- Myasthenia gravis
- Guillain-Barré syndrome

ASSESSMENT
- Patent airway
- ABG's: Low pH, high PCO_2
- Altered respiratory rate
- I&O (kidneys will compensate by getting rid of acids and saving bicarbonate)

LOC:
- CNS depression
- Drowsy
- Coma
- Vomiting
- Headache (caused by vasodilation and hypercapnia)
- Lethargic
- Confused
- Weakness
- Hypoventilation
- Dysrythmias

CLIENT NEED
Physiological Integrity

NURSING INTERVENTIONS
- Treat pain, if indicated
- Monitoring of arterial blood gases
- Adequate hydration
- Positioning for effective breathing and decreased work of breathing
- Updraft with bronchodilators
- Monitor ventilator if required
- Suction prn
- Pulmonary hygiene measures
- Administer expectorants
- O_2 (Cautiously in COPD because stimulus to breathe may be reversed)
- Percussion, postural drainage
- Administer antibiotics for respiratory infections

PATIENT TEACHING
- Pursed-lip breathing
- Effective deep breathing and coughing measures
- Quitting smoking

ASSOCIATED NURSING DIAGNOSES
- Anxiety
- Fatigue
- Pain
- Tissue perfusion, altered (cerebral)
- Airway clearance, ineffective
- Breathing pattern, ineffective
- Gas exchange, impaired
- Thought process, altered
- Ventilation, inability to sustain spontaneous

STUDY QUESTIONS

- The patient who is hypoventilating is at risk for:
  1. Pneumonia
  2. Atelectasis
  3. Respiratory alkalosis
  4. Respiratory acidosis

  Answer: 4. Respiratory acidosis

  Rationale: When respirations fall below 8-10/min., the patient is no longer blowing off CO_2 effectively. The retention of CO_2 sets up an acidotic state.

  Nursing process: Assessment

  Client need: Physiological integrity

  Clinical skill level: 2

TRACHEOSTOMY

DEFINITION
A surgical opening into the trachea in which a tube is inserted. It may be permanent or temporary.

PATHOPHYSIOLOGY
The opening is usually made at the second or third tracheal ring. An inflatable tube is inserted and held in place by tapes that fasten around the patient's neck. It is created for the purpose of maintaining oxygenation when an endotracheal tube cannot be inserted or is no longer tolerated.

ASSOCIATED MEDICAL CONDITIONS
- Laryngeal obstruction
- Burns
- Long-term ventilator management
- Facial/neck trauma
- Cancer

ASSESSMENT
- Infection
- Cuff placement
- Condition of integument around stoma
- Chest symmetry
- Breath sounds
- Respiratory distress:
  - Tachycardia
  - Tenacious secretions
  - Laryngeal stridor
  - Changes in level of consciousness
  - Restlessness
  - Increased effort to breath
- Monitor for complications:
  - Hemorrhage
  - Embolism
  - Pneumothorax
  - Aspiration
  - Subcutaneous emphysema
  - Airway obstruction (cuff protruding over tube)

- Assess need for suctioning:
  - Noisy respirations
  - Increasing restlessness
  - Increasing pulse
  - Increasing respirations
  - Non-productive cough
  - Wheezing and/or crackles
  - Patient indicates need to be suctioned
  - Aesthetics

CLIENT NEED
Physiological integrity

NURSING INTERVENTIONS
- Suction secretions prn
- Maintain humidification via trach mask
- Administer analgesics cautiously
- Provide communication techniques
- Provide alternative ways to communicate if the patient is unable to talk
- Change dressing and clean trach site daily or prn
- Suctioning should be done with caution because excessive suctioning could cause bronchospasm and damage to the tracheal mucosa and also leads to hypoxia if more than 15 seconds at a time
- Correct positioning of tube
- Continuous monitoring for signs of respiratory distress
- Pre and post oxygenate when suctioning
- Ensure that call light is within reach
- Semi-Fowler's position (facilitates ventilation and drainage, decreases strain on sutures)
- Check trach ties to make sure they are secure (Ties may become too tight due to edema)
- Monitoring of ABG's, CBC, CXR, and antibiotic therapy when there is evidence of infection

PATIENT TEACHING
- Teach care of site
- Teach patient how to communicate if patient cannot speak
- Teach patient suctioning procedures
- Avoid people with respiratory infections
- Use a humidifier at night
- Teach effective coughing and deep-breathing techniques
- Avoid use of sprays and powders
- Patient to drink up to 3 L of fluid per day to moisten secretions

ASSOCIATED NURSING DIAGNOSES
- Anxiety
- Aspiration, high risk for
- Fear
- Injury, high risk for
- Nutrition, less than body requirements, altered
- Self-care deficit: bathing/hygiene, dressing/grooming, feeding, toileting
- Airway clearance, ineffective
- Breathing pattern, ineffective
- Gas exchange, impaired
- Powerlessness
- Social isolation

STUDY QUESTIONS

■ The nurse carefully monitors the patient with a tracheostomy for adventitious breath sounds. If abnormal breath sounds are heard, the priority nursing intervention is:
1. Repositioning
2. Changing tube
3. Suctioning
4. Pain management

Answer: 3. Suctioning

Rationale: If the patient is not suctioned promptly and secretions build up, abnormal breath sounds associated with dyspnea will be heard.

Nursing process: Intervention

Client need: Physiological integrity

> Clinical skill level: 3

■ The nurse assesses airway obstruction in the patient with a tracheostomy. The first complication that she suspects is:
1. Hemorrhage
2. Embolism
3. Fistula
4. Cuff over tube

Answer: 4. Cuff over tube

Rationale: One of the most common reasons for airway obstruction in a trach patient is that the cuff is misplaced and protruding over the tube. A mucus plug from thickened secretions is also a very common cause of airway obstruction.

Nursing process: Assessment

Client need: Physiological integrity

> Clinical skill level: 3

- During the insertion of an endotracheal tube, what nursing assessment is a priority?
    1. ECG
    2. Carotid pulse
    3. Femoral pulse
    4. Vital signs

    Answer: 3. Femoral pulse

    Rationale: The femoral pulse is easily accessible and should be monitored for any irregularities during the procedure. If pulse becomes weak or absent, the physician may halt the procedure and order 100% oxygen.

    Nursing process: Assessment

    Client need: Physiological integrity

    Clinical skill level: 3

- The nursing care plan for the patient with an ET tube calls for auscultation of the lungs every hour. The nurse notes diminishing breath sounds in the left side. The nurse suspects the ET tube:
    1. Is being effective in decreasing sounds
    2. Has slipped into the right bronchus
    3. Has slipped into the left bronchus
    4. Is in the right place for maximal results

    Answer: 2. Has slipped into the right bronchus

    Rationale: Diminished or absent sounds are a cardinal sign that the tube has slipped out of place. The tube is more likely to slip into the right bronchus because it is more vertical than the left.

    Nursing process: Evaluation

    Client need: Physiological integrity

    Clinical skill level: 3

- The nursing assessment on the patient with an ET tube indicates several changes: abdominal distention, increasing dyspnea, and vomiting. The priority action is:
  1. Turn the patient over
  2. DC the ET tube
  3. Turn, cough, deep breathe
  4. Reinsert the ET tube

  Answer: 2. DC the ET tube

  Rationale: The tube may be occluding the trachea and blocking the air from entering the lungs. The tube must be removed immediately.

  Nursing process: Intervention

  Client need: Physiological integrity

  Clinical skill level: 4

TUBERCULOSIS

DEFINITION
This is a bacterial infection of the lungs. Causative agent is *Mycobacterium tuberculosis*.

PATHOPHYSIOLOGY
An inflammatory process and response of the lung macrophages to the TB bacillus. This reaction produces small, firm, white nodules known as tubercles. These tubercles can become necrotic, calcified or liquified and harbor the infective bacilli in a dormant state. If body defenses are compromised, the bacilli become active and multiply, producing an active case of the infection.

TB is a highly-communicable disease that is spread by airborne droplets. After an infected patient coughs, sneezes, laughs or even speaks, the droplets remain suspended in the air and are moved by air currents through rooms and halls. One particle of the TB organism is enough to cause infection.

ASSOCIATED MEDICAL CONDITIONS
- Pulmonary tuberculosis (TB)
- Immunocompromised conditions (HIV/CA)
- Alcoholism/malnutrition

ASSESSMENT
Initial symptoms:
- Fatigue
- Weight loss
- Anorexia
- Hemoptysis
- Pleuritic/chest pain
- Positive acid-fast bacillus test/Mantoux
- Productive cough
- Chills/sweating
- Fever
- Dyspnea
- X-ray evidence of tubercles

Breath sounds:
- Inspiratory crackles
- Bronchial wheezing

CLIENT NEED
Physiological integrity

NURSING INTERVENTIONS
- Universal precautions
- Mantoux test (0.1 ml) intradermal on inner forearm
- Wear special, particle-resistant masks
- Read Mantoux in 48-72 hours (positive if induration is 10 mm in diameter)
- Respiratory isolation
- Monitor for untoward effects of drug therapies
- Collection of sputum specimens

MEDICAL INTERVENTIONS
- Chest x-ray, especially if Mantoux is positive
- Cultures of lung tissue/fluid

Medications:
- Isoniazid (prophylaxis)
- Streptomycin
- Capreomycin
- Ethionamide
- CDC collaboration
- Provide adequate ventilation of room facility
- Ethambutol Rifampin
- Pyrazinamide
- Kanamycin

PATIENT TEACHING
- The importance of taking medications exactly as prescribed (disease will reoccur)
- Teaching patient to cover nose and mouth with disposable tissues when coughing, sneezing or laughing and placing used tissues in paper bag that can be burned.
- The importance of good handwashing after contact with body substances.

ASSOCIATED NURSING DIAGNOSES

- Activity intolerance
- Body temperature, high risk for altered
- Fear
- Noncompliance
- Family coping, compromised, ineffective
- Pain
- Hopelessness
- Home maintenance management, impaired
- Powerlessness
- Anxiety
- Breathing pattern, ineffective
- Fatigue
- Knowledge deficit
- Nutrition: less than body requirements, altered
- Social isolation
- Gas exchange, impaired
- Coping, ineffective individual

STUDY QUESTIONS

■ A patient has been exposed to tuberculosis. He has a Mantoux test. The nurse reads the test 72 hours later. Which of the following responses is interpreted as being positive?

1. Redness without induration
2. 10 mm redness
3. 5 mm redness
4. 10 mm induration

Answer: 4. 10 mm induration

Rationale: Any test result under 10 mm induration is considered inconclusive and requires the test to be given again, but at a different site. A chest x-ray may be ordered following a potentially positive test.

Nursing process: Assessment
Client need: Physiological integrity

Clinical skill level: 2

■ The patient is diagnosed as having tuberculosis. Which measure is necessary to prevent transmission of the bacilli?
1. Cover mouth when coughing
2. Use ultraviolet lights to kill the bacilli
3. Instruct others there's no need for a mask
4. Use a special mask when in the room

Answer: 4. Use a special mask when in the room

Rationale: The tubercle bacillus can penetrate an ordinary mask, and OSHA requires a special mask that cannot be easily penetrated.

Nursing process: Intervention

Client need: Physiological integrity

Clinical skill level: 2

■ The patient is being treated for tuberculosis. The nurse is teaching about the use of drug therapy and instructs the patient that:
1. He must take medication until the Mantoux is negative
2. He must take two medications instead of one
3. The typical course of treatment is a year
4. His family will need to take the medication

Answer: 2. He must take two medications instead of one

Rationale: The tubercle bacillus can develop resistance to any drug given to treat the disease. To decrease this resistance, two medications are usually prescribed. The most common medications are isoniazid and rifampin.

Nursing process: Intervention

Client need: Physiological integrity

Clinical skill level: 3

GENERAL STUDY QUESTIONS

■ Prolonged use of nasal spray for chronic sinusitis is discouraged because it:
1. Is highly addictive
2. Masks other symptoms
3. Has serious side-effects
4. Causes rebound congestion

Answer: 4. Causes rebound congestion

Rationale: Initially, the nasal spray may help the condition, but when the patient continues using it the condition becomes worse than it was in the beginning.

Nursing process: Outcome criteria

Client need: Physiological integrity

Clinical skill level: 3

■ The nurse is teaching the emphysema patient pursed-lip breathing. She explains the purpose for this is to:
1. Promote CO_2 elimination
2. Decrease coughing
3. Promote oxygen saturation
4. Promote oxygen elimination

Answer: 1. Promote CO_2 elimination

Rationale: When the patient slowly exhales, during the diaphragmatic technique that is taught in pursed-lip breathing, the expiration time is prolonged. This prolonged time allows for a greater CO_2-O_2 exchange, and the pronounced exhalation allows for greater CO_2 elimination.

Nursing process: Intervention

Client need: Physiological integrity

Clinical skill level: 2

- When there is an accumulation of secretions resulting in collapsed portions of the lung, it is documented as:
  1. Pneumothorax
  2. Hemothorax
  3. Atelectasis
  4. Pleural effusion

  Answer: 3. Atelectasis

  Rationale: Atelectasis occurs when alveoli collapse, inhibiting exchange of air. This eventually results in a shrinking, airless segment of the lung.

  Nursing process: Assessment

  Client need: Physiological integrity

  | Clinical skill level: 2 |

- A patient is suffering dyspnea. A Sengstaken-Blakemore tube is in place, and blood is in the gastric contents that are being aspirated. The nurse troubleshoots the tube by assessing:
  1. Presence of clots
  2. Esophageal secretions
  3. Tube placement
  4. Inflated balloon

  Answer: 3. Tube placement

  Rationale: The signs of dyspnea and bleeding indicate that the tube may be sliding up and partially occluding the bronchus.

  Nursing process: Assessment

  Client need: Physiological integrity

  | Clinical skill level: 3 |

- The nurse assesses soft, crackling, bubbling breath sounds that are more obvious on inspiration. This assessment should be documented as:
    1. Vesicular
    2. Bronchial
    3. Crackles
    4. Rhonchi

Answer: 3. Crackles

Rationale: Crackles can be heard upon inspiration when the small airways in the lungs contain fluid. The sound is often described as similar to the sound made by strands of hair being rubbed together.

Nursing process: Assessment

Client need: Physiological integrity

Clinical skill level: 2

- The nurse auscultates abnormal breath sounds that are high-pitched, creaking and accentuated on expiration. Which term describes this breath sound?
    1. Rhonchi
    2. Wheezes
    3. Crackles
    4. Bronchovesicular

Answer: 2. Wheezes

Rationale: Wheezing in the lungs is heard as a high-pitched, whistling sound with a prolonged inspiratory phase.

Nursing process: Assessment

Client need: Physiological integrity

Clinical skill level: 2

■ The patient is critically ill in renal failure. The nurse assesses deep, labored breaths at 44 per minute. Which term best describes this assessment?
1. Tachypnea
2. Hyperpnea
3. Cheyne-Stokes
4. Kussmaul

Answer: 4. Kussmaul
Rationale: Kussmaul, breathing is severe hyperventilation that is rapid and deep without pauses. It is associated with diabetic ketoacidosis and acidosis related to renal failure and is a compensatory mechanism to rid the body of excess acid.
Nursing process: Evaluation
Client need: Physiological integrity

Clinical skill level: 3

■ A patient who has been on the ventilator for several days is being weaned and is experiencing bronchospasm and stridor. The physician orders Dexamethasone. What is the action of this medication?
1. It is an antibiotic
2. It is a muscle relaxant
3. Decreases inflammation
4. Increases respiratory rate

Answer: 3. Decreases inflammation
Rationale: Dexamethasone is a synthetic glucocorticoid used for its anti-inflammatory properties. It will soothe irritation caused by the ET tube and decrease bronchospasm.
Nursing process: Outcome criteria
Client need: Physiological integrity

Clinical skill level: 3

- Normal lungs have the ability to stretch in order to accommodate for an increase in volume. The process is called:
    1. Pressure
    2. Compliance
    3. Resistance
    4. Exchange

    Answer: 2. Compliance

    Rationale: How the lung responds to pressure changes depends upon the mechanical properties of the lung; basically, the lungs' elasticity.

    Nursing process: Intervention

    Client need: Physiological integrity

    Clinical skill level: 2

- A patient is being prepared for a diagnostic procedure. The nurse explains, "This test allows the doctor to view your trachea and bronchi. He will insert an instrument down your throat." The nurse has partially explained a:
    1. Bronchoscopy
    2. Bronchogram
    3. Computerized tomography
    4. Pulmonary angiography

    Answer: 1. Bronchoscopy

    Rationale: This test is performed with a thin, flexible fiberoptic tube to diagnose malignancies, to remove thick secretions and foreign bodies in the bronchial tree.

    Nursing process: Intervention

    Client need: Physiological integrity

    Clinical skill level: 2

■ In teaching a respiratory patient about the process of breathing, the nurse explains that the process of external respiration occurs in the:
1. Lungs
2. Capillaries
3. Alveoli
4. Bronchioles

Answer: 3. Alveoli

Rationale: The exchange of CO_2 and O_2 in the lungs takes place in the alveoli. Internal respiration occurs the cellular level where O_2 and CO_2 are exchanged.

Nursing process: Assessment

Client need: Physiological integrity

Clinical skill level: 2

■ In assessing a patient with respiratory problems, the nurse is aware that gas exchange within the pulmonary system occurs through:
1. Osmosis
2. Diffusion
3. Active transport
4. Oncotic pressure

Answer: 2. Diffusion

Rationale: The moment of a salute from an area of higher concentration to an area of lower concentration across a semipermeable membrane is called diffusion.

Nursing process: Assessment

Client need: Physiological integrity

Clinical skill level: 2

■ Soft, rustling sounds heard primarily during inspiration over the peripheral lung fields and have a long inspiratory phase and a short expiratory phase are:
1. Adventitious
2. Bronchial
3. Vesicular
4. Bronchovesicular

Answer: 3. Vesicular

Rationale: Vesicular sounds are normal and are best heard on the periphery at the second intercostal space.

Nursing process: Assessment

Client need: Physiological integrity

Clinical skill level: 3

■ On auscultation, the nurse hears a gross, moist sound. What abnormal sound has been identified?
1. Crackles
2. Rhonchi
3. Wheeze
4. Friction rub

Answer: 2. Rhonchi

Rationale: Rhonchi is heard in conditions such as bronchitis, emphysema, pneumonia, and congestive heart failure.

Nursing process: Assessment

Client need: Physiological integrity

Clinical skill level: 3

■ Breath sounds that originate in the smaller bronchi and bronchioles that are high-pitched, sibilant and musical are called:
1. Wheezes
2. Rhonchi
3. Rales
4. Crackles

Answer: 1. Wheezes

Rationale: Wheezing is the constriction or obstruction of the pharynx, trachea, bronchi or throat.

Nursing process: Assessment

Client need: Physiological integrity

Clinical skill level: 3

■ What sound heard on auscultation is described as a grating sound, not decreased or increased after coughing is heard on both aspiration and expiration?
1. Friction rub
2. Rales
3. Rhonchi
4. Wheezes

Answer: 1. Friction rub

Rationale: A friction rub is a harsh, scratchy sound that may or may not continue when patients hold their breath.

Nursing process: Assessment

Client need: Physiological integrity

Clinical skill level: 2

- The nurse is to obtain a sputum specimen. Which instructions would result in the best specimen?
    1. "Take a deep breath. Cough. Then spit into the container."
    2. "Tomorrow you will need to collect whatever you cough up in this container."
    3. "Spit any sputum you have in your mouth into this container."
    4. "Cough and deep breathe first thing tomorrow morning and collect whatever you cough up. Now practice coughing."

    Answer: 4. "Cough and deep breathe first thing tomorrow morning and collect whatever you cough up. Now practice coughing."
    Rationale: The first sputum in the morning is important in collecting an adequate specimen for culture.
    Nursing process: Intervention
    Client need: Physiological integrity

    Clinical skill level: 2

- A patient is receiving humidified oxygen at 4 L/min via mask. The patient is taught that the purpose of humidification is:
    1. It helps lung hyperinflation
    2. It keeps the airways moist
    3. It maintains a systemic hydration
    4. It promotes gas exchange

    Answer: 2. It keeps the airways moist
    Rationale: O_2 that is not humidified is very drying, and can promote infection.
    Nursing process: Intervention
    Client need: Physiological integrity

    Clinical skill level: 2

■ Which nursing interventions are planned for the patient who has a nasal cannula in place?
1. Assess nares for skin breakdown every 6 hours
2. Check the patency of the cannula every 2 hours
3. Inspect the mouth every 6 hours
4. Secure the cannula to the nose with non-allergenic tape

Answer: 1. Assess nares for skin breakdown every 6 hours

Rationale: The nasal cannula is constantly rubbing at the patient's face and ears, and breakdown can occur within a few hours once irritation begins.

Nursing process: Intervention

Client need: Physiological integrity

Clinical skill level: 2

■ The nurse is assessing a 64-year-old man. Which assessment is an abnormal finding upon inspection?
1. Inspiration/expiration ratio of 1:2
2. Leans forward with hands on knees
3. Skin translucent, mucus membranes moist
4. Quiet respirations at rate of 20

Answer: 2. Leans forward with hands on knees

Rationale: The older person who suffers respiratory problems, such as COPD, tends to lean forward.

Nursing process: Assessment

Client need: Physiological integrity

Clinical skill level: 2

■ A patient is scheduled for a bronchoscopy and bronchogram. After signing the permit, the patient asks if the procedure will be painful. The best response is:
1. "Don't worry about it. Your doctor knows what he is doing."
2. "There will be some discomfort but you will be given medications."
3. "It won't be anything you can't tolerate."
4. "No, it doesn't hurt. You won't feel a thing."

Answer: 2. "There will be some discomfort but you will be given medications."

Rationale: The physician will prescribe a sedative or narcotic prior to this invasive procedure.

Nursing process: Intervention

Client need: Physiological integrity

Clinical skill level: 2

■ Following the bronchoscopy, the patient complains of thirst. The nurse:
1. Checks for diet order on the chart
2. Checks for the gag reflex
3. Tells the patient to wait 8 hours
4. Proceeds to give ice chips slowly

Answer: 2. Checks for the gag reflex

Rationale: Before the patient is given fluids, the nurse must make sure he can swallow. If the gag reflex is not intact, the patient may aspirate, and this would cause dangerous complications.

Nursing process: Assessment

Client need: Physiological integrity

Clinical skill level: 2

UNIT 2

CARDIOVASCULAR SYSTEM

- Angina Pectoris
- Cardiac Failure
  - Left-Sided Failure
  - Right-Sided Failure
- Congestive Heart Failure
- Hypertension
- Myocardial Infarction
- Pulmonary Edema

ANGINA PECTORIS

DEFINITION
Angina pectoris is a symptom characterized by discomfort in the chest. It is caused by inadequate blood supply to the myocardium.

PATHOPHYSIOLOGY
Myocardial ischemia is caused primarily by an inadequate blood supply or an increased demand for oxygen. The symptoms of angina differs from myocardial infarction in that angina is relieved by nitroglycerin and MI is not.

ASSOCIATED MEDICAL CONDITIONS
Myocardial infarction

ASSESSMENT:
- Discomfort in chest:
  - Aching
  - Tightness
  - Heaviness
  - Dull Pain
- Hypotension
- Tachycardia
- Activity or exertion
- Hypertension
- Circulatory status

CLIENT NEED:
Physiological integrity

NURSING INTERVENTIONS
- Identify exact site of distress
- Administer nitroglycerin
- Encourage deep breathing to induce relaxation
- Monitor length of time (if not relieved in 15 minutes, other problems should be considered)

PATIENT TEACHING
- Teach precipitating factors:
  - Exercise
  - Emotional stress
  - Eating heavy meal
  - Exposure to cold

ASSOCIATED NURSING DIAGNOSES
- Activity intolerance, high risk for
- Anxiety
- Cardiac output, decreased
- Gas exchange, impaired
- Injury, high risk for
- Powerlessness
- Coping, ineffective individual
- Fear
- Breathing pattern, ineffective
- Hopelessness
- Pain

STUDY QUESTIONS

■ During the nursing assessment, the nurse finds that a 59-year-old patient has a history of angina and has been prescribed nitroglycerin. This drug is used for its action as a/an:
1. Analgesic
2. Vasoconstrictor
3. Vasodilator
4. Antihypertensive

Answer: 3. Vasodilator

Rationale: Nitroglycerin dilates the coronary arteries allowing for oxygenation of the myocardial tissue, and relieving the pain and reducing preload.

Nursing process: Outcome criteria

Client need: Physiological integrity

> Clinical skill level: 3

■ Patient education regarding nitroglycerin should emphasize that:
1. New tablets should be obtained every year
2. Side effects of hypotension and headache are common
3. Tablets might cause tingling if they have lost potency
4. Hypertension may result from prolonged use

Answer: 2. Side effects of hypotension and headache are common

Rationale: Because nitroglycerin may dilate vessels very quickly, the side effect of this is hypotension, and headache.

Nursing process: Intervention

Client need: Physiological integrity

Clinical skill level: 3

■ The pain of angina pectoris is the result of:
1. Decreased contractility
2. Decreasing cardiac output
3. Inadequate coronary blood flow
4. Decreasing stroke volume

Answer: 3. Inadequate coronary blood flow

Rationale: When myocardial tissue is not adequately oxygenated, the resulting ischemia causes this discomfort.

Nursing process: Assessment

Client need: Physiological integrity

Clinical skill level: 3

- A patient is experiencing angina. What does the nurse assess?
    1. Pain that requires narcotics
    2. Pain that lasts 30 minutes
    3. Unrelenting pain that will not stop
    4. Pain relieved by bedrest

    Answer: 4. Pain relieved by bedrest

    Rationale: Angina is relieved by rest and nitroglycerin. The pain of myocardial infarction is not relieved except with narcotics. Pain that is relieved is angina; pain that is not relieved could signal an MI.

    Nursing process:

    Client need: Physiological integrity

    Clinical skill level: 3

- Nitroglycerin is placed at the patient's bedside. The nurse explains to the patient that this drug:
    1. Increases contractility
    2. Increases the heart rate
    3. Decreases contractility
    4. Decreases venous return

    Answer: 4. Decreases venous return

    Rationale: The drug not only dilates the coronary arteries, but causes a peripheral vasodilation, which decreases venous return. Therefore, the heart does not have to work as hard and there is less oxygen consumption. As a vasodilator, this medication causes peripheral as well as coronary vasodilation. Because venous return is decreased, the heart doesn't have to work so hard against the resistance.

    Nursing process: Outcome criteria

    Client need: Physiological integrity

    Clinical skill level: 2

CARDIAC FAILURE
LEFT-SIDED

DEFINITION
In left-sided failure, the ventricle cannot eject all of the blood effectively. As a result, pressure builds up in the left atrium and backs up into the pulmonary veins and pulmonary capillaries.

PATHOPHYSIOLOGY
When the hydrostatic pressure in the pulmonary capillaries rises, fluid moves into the interstitial spaces from the general circulation and, eventually, into the alveoli causing pulmonary edema. Left-sided cardiac failure is primarily caused by hypertension and ischemic heart disease.

ASSOCIATED MEDICAL CONDITIONS
Myocardial Infarction

ASSESSMENT
- Early signs:
  - Weakness
  - Fatigue
  - Difficulty concentrating
  - Palpitations
  - Anxiety
  - Low tolerance for activity or exercise
- Dyspnea
  - Shallow respirations
  - Tachypnea
  - Use of accessory muscles
  - At first, upon exertion
  - Later stages, at rest
- Dry, hacking cough
- Pulsus aternans
- Cyanosis
- Tachycardia
- Orthopnea
- Crackles
- S_3 and S_4 (gallop rhythms)
- Cardiac dysrhythmias

- Cheyne-Stokes respirations
- Paroxysmal nocturnal dyspnea

CLIENT NEED
- Physiological integrity

NURSING INTERVENTIONS
- Monitor ABGs
- Place in semi or high Fowler's
- Monitor ECG
- Observe for cardiogenic shock

PATIENT TEACHING
- Teach low-salt diet
- Teach the importance of taking diuretics at times prescribed, especially in avoiding increased nocturia

ASSOCIATED NURSING DIAGNOSES
- Fatigue
- Fear
- Activity intolerance, high risk for
- Cardiac output, decreased
- Gas exchange, impaired

STUDY QUESTIONS

■ S_3 with gallop rhythm is indicative of:
1. Right-sided heart failure
2. Normal heart sound at S_3
3. Left ventricular failure
4. Extensive myocardial damage

Answer: 3. Left ventricular failure

Rationale: In adults, S_3 is an abnormal sound indicative of left ventricular failure. S_3 is considered normal in children.

Nursing process: Assessment

Client need: Physiological integrity

Clinical skill level: 3

■ A patient is suffering left ventricular failure. Which assessment is indicative of this complication?
1. Low blood pressure
2. Edema in left arm
3. Orthopnea
4. Pulsating neck veins

Answer: 3. Orthopnea

Rationale: The patient with left-sided failure has dyspnea when lying down because the left ventricle cannot empty completely when fluid from the extremities flows back to the pulmonary circulation.

Nursing process: Assessment

Client need: Physiological integrity

Clinical skill level: 2

■ During a cardiac assessment the nurse hears a third heart sound (S_3). This is documented as a:
1. Atrial gallop
2. Aortic gallop
3. Systolic gallop
4. Ventricular gallop

Answer: 4. Ventricular gallop

Rationale: A third heart sound is known as a ventricular gallop. It is a low-pitched sound that immediately follows the second heart sound (S_2).

Nursing process: Assessment

Client need: Physiological integrity

Clinical skill level: 3

CARDIAC FAILURE RIGHT-SIDED

DEFINITION
Failure of the right ventricle results in an accumulation of blood in peripheral tissues and abdominal organs. Right-sided failure is called cor pulmonale (or pulmonary heart disease) when the underlying cause is pulmonary disease.

PATHOPHYSIOLOGY
Right-sided failure often ensues left-sided failure. An overload of blood in systemic veins causes high venous pressure and edema.

ASSOCIATED MEDICAL CONDITIONS
- Congestive Heart Failure
- Pulmonary Edema

ASSESSMENT
- Hepatic enlargement
- Peripheral edema
- Anorexia
- In late stages, ascites
- Jugular venous distentions (indicating elevated venous pressure)
- Fatigue
- Nausea
- Abdominal distention
- Nocturia

CLIENT NEED
Physiological integrity

NURSING INTERVENTIONS
- Encourage bedrest
- Monitor ECG
- Monitor ABGs
- Strict I&O
- Restrict salt to 2-3 g/day
- Administer diuretics

- Observe water restriction if ordered
- Monitor PT time (increase indicative of cardiomegaly)

PATIENT TEACHING
- Teach low salt diet
- Teach the importance of taking diuretics at times prescribed, especially in avoiding increased nocturia

ASSOCIATED NURSING DIAGNOSES
- Activity intolerance
- Cardiac output, decreased
- Fatigue
- Hopelessness
- Powerlessness
- Sleep pattern disturbance
- Anxiety
- Coping, ineffective individual
- Fear
- Noncompliance: diet
- Role performance, altered
- Urinary elimination, altered

STUDY QUESTIONS

■ The drug of choice in the treatment of a cardiac patient when the goal is to increase the contractibility of the heart is:
1. Inderal
2. Digitalis
3. Vasopressors
4. Coumadin

Answer: 2. Digitalis

Rationale: The most commonly-prescribed digitalis, Lanoxin, is an antiarrhythmic that strengthens the force of contraction of the heart muscle.

Nursing process: Intervention

Client need: Physiological integrity

Clinical skill level: 2

■ With rising CVP the nurse would suspect:
1. Fluid volume excess
2. Myocardial infarction
3. Hypovolemic shock
4. Pulmonary edema

Answer: 1. Fluid volume excess

Rationale: CVP is a measure of circulating blood and is reflective of right ventricular function. Since right ventricular failure is often secondary to left ventricular failure, a rising CVP is a late sign of left ventricular failure.

Nursing process: Assessment

Client need: Physiological integrity

Clinical skill level: 3

CONGESTIVE HEART FAILURE

DEFINITION
The term congestive heart failure is synonymous with cardiac failure. It implies the combined effects of left-sided and right-sided failure.

PATHOPHYSIOLOGY
A number of factors can contribute to cardiac failure. However, primarily, it is the result of myocardial tissue damage in which stroke volume (SV) and heart rate (HR) are impaired, eventually shutting down cardiac output (CO).

ASSOCIATED MEDICAL CONDITIONS
- Pneumonia
- Pulmonary embolism
- Chronic obstructive pulmonary disease

ASSESSMENT
- Dyspnea upon exertion
- Orthopnea
- Chest pain
- Peripheral edema
- Distended neck veins
- Fatigue
- Paroxysmal nocturnal dyspnea
- Signs and symptoms of pulmonary edema:
  - Pink, frothy sputum
  - Respiratory distress
  - Wheezing
  - Coughing
  - Orthopnea
  - Diaphoresis
  - Cyanosis
  - Cold, clammy extremities

CLIENT NEED
Physiological integrity

NURSING INTERVENTIONS
- Encourage salt restriction to 2-3 g/day
- Restrict fluid as ordered
- IV at KVO only
- Monitor Swan-Ganz catheter
- Place in high-Fowler's position
- Strict I&O
- Administer O_2
- Monitor for cardiogenic shock

PATIENT TEACHING
- Teach low-salt diet
- Teach the importance of taking diuretics at times prescribed, especially in avoiding increased nocturia

ASSOCIATED NURSING DIAGNOSES
- Cardiac output, decreased
- Anxiety
- Fear
- Hopelessness
- Pain
- Spiritual distress: distress of the human spirit
- Activity intolerance, high risk for
- Fatigue
- Gas exchange, impaired
- Noncompliance: diet
- Powerlessness
- Tissue perfusion: renal, cardiopulmonary

STUDY QUESTIONS

■ A patient is admitted through the emergency room for congestive heart failure. Shortly after admission, the nurse assesses his condition. He is dyspneic and slightly cyanotic. Nursing action is to:
1. Call the doctor
2. Start the oxygen
3. Elevate the head of the bed
4. Start an IV

Answer: 2. Start the oxygen
Rationale: The dyspnea and cyanosis indicate body tissues are not being oxygenated, and O_2 must be administered.
Nursing process: Intervention
Client need: Physiological integrity

> Clinical skill level: 2

■ Congestive heart failure can be evaluated through the use of a:
1. CVP into the left atrium
2. Swan-Ganz catheter in the pulmonary artery
3. Pulmonary artery (wedge) pressure line into the left atrium
4. Pulmonary venous catheter in the right atrium

Answer: 2. Swan-Ganz catheter in the pulmonary artery
Rationale: The Swan-Ganz is a balloon-tipped catheter that is threaded through the right atrium and ventricle, and into the pulmonary artery. The purpose is to measure pulmonary artery pressure and pulmonary capillary wedge pressure. These readings give precise indications of circulating volume and pulmonary status.
Nursing process: Evaluation
Client need: Physiological integrity

> Clinical skill level: 3

■ The presence of an S3 heart sound indicates:
1. A normal finding in an adult
2. A split sound produced by the atrial valve
3. Pulmonary embolism
4. Impending congestive heart failure

Answer: 4. Impending congestive heart failure

Rationale: The S3 is an early diastolic sound that is abnormal in the adult and normal in a child. The sound indicates a decreased compliance of the ventricle and heard in patients with MI and CHF.

Nursing process: Assessment

Client need: Physiological integrity

Clinical skill level: 3

HYPERTENSION

DEFINITION
Hypertension is a condition of persistent elevation of systolic pressure above 160 mm Hg and diastolic pressure above 90 mm Hg. The blood pressure exceeds 140/90 on at least two consecutive readings.

PATHOPHYSIOLOGY
Blood pressure equals cardiac output times peripheral resistance. (BP = CO × PR) For essential hypertension to occur, one or more of the following conditions must be present: 1. arteriolar alterations, 2. Changes in sympathetic role, 3. Hormonal influences and or genetic factors.

Cardiac output is best measured by systolic pressure and peripheral resistance is best revealed in the diastolic pressure. In addition, some forms of hypertension are the consequence of an underlying disease process.

ASSOCIATED MEDICAL CONDITIONS
- Atherosclerosis
- Renal disease
- Aldosteronism
- Diabetes mellitus
- Malignant hypertension
- Cardiac hypertrophy
- Pheochromocytoma
- Myocardial infarction

ASSESSMENT
- Systolic blood pressure
- Dietary habits
- Knowledge of nutrition
- Medications prescribed for hypertension
- Highest known pressure
- History of epistaxis
- Race
- Sex
- Family history of hypertension
- Diastolic blood pressure
- Weight and height
- Usual pressure reading
- Occipital headache, especially in the morning
- Stressors and coping strategies
- Level of anxiety
- Smoking
- Obesity
- Pulse pressure (difference between the systolic and diastolic)

CLIENT NEED
Physiological integrity

NURSING INTERVENTIONS
- Patient teaching and counseling R/T risk factors, dietary modifications, medication regimen and health maintenance
- Exercise program
- Administer antihypertensive medication—monotherapy progressing to multitherapy as indicated.

PATIENT TEACHING
- Maintain ideal weight
- Relaxation techniques
- Adhere to salt-restricted diet (2-3 gm/day)
- Establish a daily exercise routine
- Quit smoking cigarettes
- Maintaining sexual function
- If obese, reduce weight (weight loss decreases diastolic pressure)
- Alcohol intake should be restricted (Amounts that exceed 2 oz. of 100-proof whiskey, 8 oz. wine, or 24 oz. beer daily is considered excessive)

ASSOCIATED NURSING DIAGNOSES
- Anxiety
- Fatigue
- Gas exchange, impaired
- Cardiac output, decreased
- Alteration in sexual function
- Tissue perfusion, altered: renal, cerebral, cardiopulmonary, peripheral
- Denial, ineffective coping
- Fear
- Hopelessness
- Activity intolerance, high risk for
- Altered health maintenance R/T knowledge deficit

STUDY QUESTIONS

■ A 57-year-old woman has her blood pressure checked at a health fair. Her reading is 186/94. The most appropriate response to this finding would be to tell the patient:
1. That she has hypertension and should see her doctor immediately
2. Everything is fine and quietly suggest to her daughter that her mother should have medical attention
3. That her blood pressure is about normal for her age
4. That her blood pressure is elevated and recommend further evaluation

Answer: 4. That her blood pressure is elevated and recommend further evaluation

Rationale: The highest reading within normal limits is 140/90. Her BP requires further evaluation by a physician.

Nursing process: Intervention

Client need: Physiological integrity

Clinical skill level: 2

■ Which of the following is a sign of portal hypertension?
1. Left-side pain
2. Right-side pain
3. GI bleeding
4. Productive cough

Answer: 3. GI bleeding

Rationale: Varicosities caused by the increased pressures throughout the portal system may rupture and hemorrhage in the GI tract and rectum.

Nursing process: Assessment

Client need: Physiological integrity

Clinical skill level: 2

MYOCARDIAL INFARCTION

DEFINITION
Myocardial infarction occurs when a part of the myocardium becomes ischemic and, eventually, necrosis causes a sudden interruption to coronary blood flow. When necrosis occurs, contraction in that part of the heart stops.

ASSOCIATED MEDICAL CONDITIONS
- Heart attack
- Coronary occlusion
- Cardiogenic shock
- Congestive heart failure
- Coronary thrombosis

ASSESSMENT
- Hypotension
- Severe chest pain:
  - Substernal
  - Described as crushing, squeezing pressures
  - Lasts longer than 15 minutes
  - Unrelieved by nitroglycerin
  - Radiates to left arm, shoulder, jaw
- Signs of cardiogenic shock:
  - Dysrhythmias
  - Low blood pressure
  - Weak, rapid pulse
  - Confusion and agitation (due to cerebral hypoxia)
  - Urinary output   ml/hour for two hour period
  - Cold, clammy skin
  - No relief of symptoms with administration of analgesic and oxygen
- Nausea and vomiting
- Level of anxiety
- Skin cold, clammy, gray in color
- Cyanosis in nailbeds, tip of nose, earlobes, or extremities
- Diaphoresis
- Peripheral pulses
- Abdominal pain, often described as indigestion

CLIENT NEED
Physiological integrity

NURSING INTERVENTIONS
- Start IV stat (for administration of emergency medications)
- Monitor ECG
- Ensure blood drawn for cardiac enzyme studies
- Provide emotional support to decrease anxiety and allay fear
- Monitor ABGs
- Administer morphine IV stat (pain relief is the priority intervention to stop recurring attacks)

PATIENT TEACHING
- Stop smoking cigarettes
- Adhere to exercise regimen, emphasizing aerobic exercise
- Encourage low-fat diet
- Encourage weight loss, if appropriate

STUDY QUESTIONS

■ A patient complains of sharp pain in the chest and down his left arm. This pain is documented as:
1. Recurring pain
2. Displaced pain
3. Radiating pain
4. Radiohumeral pain

Answer: 3. Radiating pain

Rationale: Pain often radiates from the source of the discomfort. Chest pain that radiates down the left arm may signal an MI.

Nursing process: Assessment

Client need: Physiological integrity

Clinical skill level: 2

■ A patient is admitted to the emergency room with severe chest pain. He is short of breath, restless, apprehensive, pale, and diaphoretic. The pain is substernal and radiates to the jaw and left arm. The initial intervention is:
1. Have him lie down flat
2. Administer oxygen and start IV
3. Have him lie in a semi-Fowler's position
4. Administer pain medication stat

Answer: 2. Administer oxygen and start IV

Rationale: This patient may be having a heart attack. O_2 is required to keep tissues oxygenated, and access IV is required to administer emergency medications.

Nursing process: Intervention

Client need: Physiological integrity

Clinical skill level: 3

■ The physician orders several lab tests for the MI patient, when the test results are returned, the nurse recognizes the most reliable indicator of a myocardial infarction is:
1. LDH
2. ECG
3. CK
4. CK-MB

Answer: 4. CK-MB

Rationale: Creatine kinase (CK) and the isoenzyme that is specific for the cardiac tissue, CK-MB, is the most specific test in diagnosing a heart attack. CK-MB is elevated within 2-4 hours of an MI.

Nursing process: Evaluation

Client need: Physiological integrity

Clinical skill level: 3

■ The primary reason IM injections are not given post-MI is because the injection may alter:
1. Pain threshold
2. Pain tolerance
3. Serum enzyme readings
4. T-wave readings

Answer: 3. Serum enzyme readings

Rationale: An injection of morphine IM may falsely elevate the cardiac enzymes that are being evaluated when the physician is in the process of diagnosing an MI.

Nursing process: Outcome criteria

Client need: Physiological integrity

Clinical skill level: 3

■ The nurse is closely monitoring the MI patient. The nurse is aware that hypotension is a warning sign of:
1. Pulmonary edema
2. Cardiac shock
3. Fatal dysrhythmias
4. Another heart attack

Answer: 2. Cardiac shock

Rationale: Falling blood pressure is an early warning of shock and is due to the decreased ability of the failing heart to produce adequate cardiac output.

Nursing process: Assessment

Client need: Physiological integrity

Clinical skill level: 2

- The plan of care for the MI patient should include:
  1. Encouraging patient to eat bland foods
  2. Turning off noisy stimuli
  3. Limiting food and fluids
  4. Avoiding rectal temperatures

  Answer: 4. Avoiding rectal temperatures
  Rationale: Rectal stimulation may cause the vagal nerve to react, increasing heart activity and myocardial oxygen demand.
  Nursing process: Intervention
  Client need: Physiological integrity

  Clinical skill level: 2

- Nursing priorities the first 24-72 hours following an MI are:
  1. Supportive therapy, coping efforts and minimizing activity
  2. Decreasing anxiety and fostering dependence
  3. Strict I & O and ABG interpretation
  4. Implement orders and regulate HBGs

  Answer: 1. Supportive therapy, coping efforts and minimizing activity
  Rationale: Rest is necessary for reduction of cardiac output. Sedatives and antianxiety agents are often prescribed to help the patient relax.
  Nursing process: Intervention
  Client need: Physiological integrity

  Clinical skill level: 3

- A patient is 24 hours post-MI. His temperature is 101.2 degrees. The nurse evaluates this as:
  1. An infection
  2. Congestive heart failure
  3. A normal response to MI
  4. Possible pericarditis

  Answer: 3. A normal response to MI

  Rationale: An increase in temperature is the normal inflammatory response to tissue destruction. It occurs 24 to 48 hours post infarction.

  Nursing process: Evaluation

  Client need: Physiological integrity

  Clinical skill level: 3

- Because of the tissue and cell damage following an MI, the nurse anticipates finding:
  1. An increased K+ level
  2. A decreased K+ level
  3. An increased Na level
  4. A decreased Na level

  Answer: 1. An increased K+ level

  Rationale: Potassium, an intracellular ion, is released into the extracellular space during cell destruction and the serum level goes up.

  Nursing process: Evaluation

  Client need: Physiological integrity

  Clinical skill level: 3

PULMONARY EDEMA

DEFINITION
The abnormal accumulation of fluid or blood in the lungs.

PATHOPHYSIOLOGY
There is more blood in the pulmonary vascular system that is being delivered by the right ventricle than the left ventricle can accommodate. The development of pulmonary edema signals that ventricular function has become inadequate and cardiac failure may be imminent.

ASSOCIATED MEDICAL DIAGNOSES
- Cardiac: Atherosclerosis, hypertension, acute MI with left ventricular failure
- Rapid administration of intravenous fluids
- Noncardiac: Toxic inhalants, drug overdose, smoke inhalation

ASSESSMENT
- Dramatic dyspnea
- Restlessness
- Cold moist hands
- Grayish skin-pallor
- Confusion
- Orthopnea
- Tachycardia with weak pulse
- Production cough of frothy fluid tinged with blood
- Hypoxia
- Insomnia
- Cyanosis
- Distended neck veins
- Stupor
- Audible wheezing
- Anxiety may develop into panic

CLIENT NEED
Physiological integrity

NURSING INTERVENTIONS

- Monitor ABGs to assess oxygenation
- Monitor for fluid and electrolyte imbalances
- Endotracheal intubation
- Administer Morphine to reduce anxiety, respiratory rate, decrease peripheral resistance, dilate venous circulation
- Conserve energy by limiting activity and assessing ADLs
- Administer Lasix to draw off fluids
- Administer O_2 to relieve hypoxia and dyspnea
- Inotropic drugs, i.e. dobutamine, amrinone, nitro
- Mechanical ventilation (positive and expiratory pressure [PEEP] reduces venous return, lowers pulmonary capillary pressure and increases oxygenation)

PATIENT TEACHING

- Monitoring of signs and symptoms R/T untoward effects of drug therapy.
- Dietary modifications

ASSOCIATED NURSING DIAGNOSES

- Anxiety
- Hopelessness
- Powerlessness
- Breathing pattern, ineffective
- Tissue perfusion, altered (cerebral, cardiopulmonary)
- Fear
- Hyperthermia
- Gas exchange: impaired
- Ventilation, inability to sustain spontaneous
- Altered health maintenance R/T knowledge deficit regarding dietary modifications

STUDY QUESTIONS

■ Pulmonary edema would indicate the patient is suffering:
1. Hypovolemic shock
2. Left ventricular failure
3. Renal failure
4. Vasogenic shock

Answer: 2. Left ventricular failure

Rationale: The accumulation of fluid in the lungs may be caused by several conditions including, congestive heart failure, cardiogenic shock, and drug overdose.

Nursing process: Assessment

Client need: Physiological integrity

Clinical skill level: 3

■ The first sign of pulmonary edema is:
1. Pallor
2. Restlessness
3. Falling blood pressure
4. Decreasing pulse pressure

Answer: 2. Restlessness

Rationale: During the initial onset of pulmonary edema, the pulmonary vessels fill with fluid and begin to leak. The patient may not be aware of what is happening, but will respond to the subtle changes with restlessness and anxiety. Then, dyspnea hits suddenly and the signs become obvious.

Nursing process: Evaluation

Client need: Physiological integrity

Clinical skill level: 2

■ Fresh-water drowning and salt-water drowning have dramatically different effects upon the lungs. However, they both have the same deadly outcome, which is:
1. Collapsed lungs
2. Pulmonary edema
3. O_2-Co_2 shift
4. Sudden hypotensive crisis

Answer: 2. Pulmonary edema

Rationale: The hyperosmolar effect of salt water pulls massive amounts of water into the alveoli. In fresh-water drowning, surfactant is washed out by the fresh water, forcing the collapse of the alveoli. The alveoli then fill with water. Either way, the alveoli fill up, and the fatal result is pulmonary edema.

Nursing process: Evaluation

Client need: Physiological integrity

Clinical skill level: 3

General Study Questions

■ IV fluids may be restricted after cardiac surgery. The rationale for this is to:
1. Stabilize blood pressure
2. Decrease workload on heart
3. Decrease workload on renal system
4. Decrease risk of pulmonary embolism

Answer: 2. Decrease workload on heart

Rationale: Increased fluids will increase the workload on the heart. If there is a dramatic increase in fluid volume, such as IV administration, the heart's workload will increase.

Nursing process: Outcome criteria

Client need: Physiological integrity

Clinical skill level: 3

- Anticholinesterase drugs can cause side effects such as bradycardia. If this happens the nurse prepares to give:
  1. Calan
  2. Atropine
  3. Neostigmine
  4. Vasopressin

  Answer: 2. Atropine

  Rationale: Atropine blocks vagal impulses to the heart, increasing heart rate, and is often prescribed in bradycardia.

  Nursing process: Evaluation

  Client need: Physiological integrity

  Clinical skill level: 3

- A calcium channel blocker is prescribed to a cardiac patient. During patient teaching the nurse describes the action of the drug as:
  1. Increasing arterial pressure
  2. Increasing atrial pressure
  3. Reducing the work load of the ventricle
  4. Reducing dilation of coronary arteries

  Answer: 3. Reducing the work load of the ventricle

  Rationale: Medications such as diltiazem (Cardizem), nifedipine (Procardia), and verapamil (Calan) decrease myocardial contractility, thereby decreasing the O_2 demand and workload of the heart.

  Nursing process: Intervention

  Client need: Physiological integrity

  Clinical skill level: 2

■ The most common time for naturally-occurring death is:
1. 2 a.m.
2. 6 a.m.
3. 11 a.m.
4. 8 p.m.

Answer: 2. 6 a.m.

Rationale: Research indicates that cardiovascular morbidity and morality peak in the morning according to a circadian variation.

Nursing process: Assessment

Client need: Physiological integrity

Clinical skill level: 2

■ The nurse is assessing for pericardial friction rub in the patient diagnosed with pericarditis. She asks the patient to:
1. Stand up and breathe deeply
2. Sit up and lean forward
3. Sit up and lean to the side
4. Lie on side and breathe normally

Answer: 2. Sit up and lean forward

Rationale: Pericardial friction rub is an abnormal breath sound best heard when the patient is sitting up and leaning forward at the fifth intercostal space during systole. Other signs of pericarditis are fever, tachycardia, dyspnea and chest pain.

Nursing process: Assessment

Client need: Physiological integrity

Clinical skill level: 3

- The patient with pericarditis complains of sharp chest pain. Patient teaching should emphasize that the patient:
    1. Sit upright
    2. Lean forward
    3. Stand up
    4. Lie flat

    Answer: 1. Sit upright

    Rationale: The chest pain associated with pericarditis is often relieved with the patient sits upright.

    Nursing process: Intervention

    Client need: Physiological integrity

    | Clinical skill level: 3 |

- In assessing a patient for cardiac problems, the nurse listens to the point of maximal impulse. It is located:
    1. At the 3rd intercostal space near the apex
    2. At the 4th intercostal space near the apex
    3. At the 5th intercostal space near the apex
    4. Between the nipple and midsternal line

    Answer: 3. At the 5th intercostal space near the apex

    Rationale: This area, called the PMI is the spot where, usually, the heart beat is heard most distinctly.

    Nursing process: Assessment

    Client need: Physiological integrity

    | Clinical skill level: 1 |

UNIT 3
IMMUNE SYSTEM

- Acquired Immunodeficiency Syndrome (AIDS)
- Anaphylaxis
- Infection
- Systemic Lupus Erythematosus (SLE)

AIDS

ACQUIRED IMMUNODEFICIENCY SYNDROME

DEFINITION
The Centers for Disease Control (CDC) has a complex definition of AIDS that generally states "a case of AIDS is defined as an illness characterized by one or more of the following indicator diseases, depending on the status of laboratory evidence of HIV infection." (See list of diagnoses below)

PATHOPHYSIOLOGY
The human immunodeficiency virus (HIV) is the causative agent. Once HIV infects the bloodstream, it invades helper T lymphocytes, and with reverse transcriptase it converts RNA into DNA and incorporates it into the host cell's genetic material. Once immunologically stimulated, the infected cell reproduces the virus and dies in the process.

ASSOCIATED MEDICAL CONDITIONS

- *Pneumocystis carinii* pneumonia
- Herpes simplex, zoster
- Cervical cancer
- Cytomegalovirus
- Lymphoma of the brain
- Candidiasis of esophagus, vagina, integument, lungs, trachea
- Toxoplasmosis of the brain
- Herpes simplex virus infection that persists for more than one month
- Lymphoid interstitial pneumonia
- Cryptococcus neoformans
- Histoplasmosis
- Kaposi's sarcoma
- Mycobacterium avium complex
- Cryptosporidiosis (with explosive diarrhea) that persists for more than one month
- Multifaceted leukoencephalopathy
- Tuberculosis

ASSESSMENT

- Weight loss
- Lymphadenopathy
- Explosive, uncontrollable diarrhea
- Dry cough
- Dehydration
- Candida infections
- Fear
- Fever (usually of unknown origin)
- Weakness
- Fatigue
- Productive cough (with pneumonia)
- Depression
- Kaposi's sarcoma
- Hairy leukoplakia
- Anxiety
- Signs of dementia: confusion, disorientation, psychosis

With cryptococcal meningitis:

- Photophobia
- Headaches
- Distorted vision
- Mood swings
- Hallucinations
- Blindness

CLIENT NEED

Physiological integrity

NURSING INTERVENTIONS

- Universal precautions
- Force fluids
- Monitor electrolytes
- Provide skin care
- Change linens prn when suffering fever and chills
- Educate patient regarding self-care
- Keep lesions clean and dry
- Wipe up blood spills with 1:10 solution of bleach and water
- Weigh daily
- Scrupulous handwashing
- Monitor I & O
- Monitor temperature
- Offer supportive therapy; especially related to grieving and social isolation
- Provide high-calorie nutrition
- Offer saline mouthwash frequently
- Towel patient with 1:10 solution of isopropyl alcohol and water to clear and dry skin during night sweats

MEDICAL INTERVENTIONS
- Order ELISA (to detect antibodies) CD_4 and CD_8 counts
- Order Western blot test (to confirm presence of HIV)
- Prescribe zidovadine (Retrovir, AZT) — decreases HIV and improves immune functioning
- Prescribe Thrimethoprim (for *Pneumocystis carinii* pneumonia)
- Prescribe Amphotericin B (Fungizone) — for candida and cryptococcal infections
- Ventilator management
- Nutritional support—TPN

PATIENT TEACHING
- Universal precautions at home
- Name and telephone number of support group
- Adequate nutritional needs
- Assess daily for signs/symptoms of infection:
  - Temperature check,
  - Thrush,
  - Candida,
  - Herpes
- Educate regarding high risk behaviors
- Avoidance of situations with high infection potential, i.e. children, crowds

ASSOCIATED NURSING DIAGNOSES
- Anxiety
- Diarrhea
- Coping, ineffective individual
- Grieving, dysfunctional
- Powerlessness
- Knowledge deficit
- Nutrition, less than body requirements, altered
- Skin integrity, impaired
- Powerlessness
- Fear
- Fatigue
- Body temperature, high risk for altered
- Hopelessness: suicidal ideation
- Infection, high risk for
- Social isolation
- Management of therapeutic regime, ineffective
- Spiritual distress
- Thought processes, altered

STUDY QUESTIONS

■ A 22-year-old IV drug user has been diagnosed with AIDS. He has been admitted to the hospital with pneumocystis pneumonia. An essential part of the care plan includes:
1. Strict isolation
2. Universal precautions
3. Respiratory isolation
4. Reverse isolation

Answer: 2. Universal precautions

Rationale: Universal precautions are required for ALL patients in the hospital. The concern about transmission of AIDS is one of the major reasons the CDC recommends it, and OSHA requires it.

Nursing process: Implementation

Client need: Physiological integrity

> Clinical skill level: 2

■ The nurse assesses a reddish-purple lesion on the AIDS patient's wrist. She evaluates this as:
1. Malignant melanoma
2. Ulceration of AIDS
3. Basal cell carcinoma
4. Kaposi's sarcoma

Answer: 4. Kaposi's sarcoma

Rationale: One of the first signs of AIDS in the early '80s was the appearance of KS among people who were dying of a mysterious illness — AIDS.

Nursing process: Assessment

Client need: Physiological integrity

> Clinical skill level: 2

- A pregnant patient, 26, is admitted with a productive cough, diarrhea, night sweats, and generalized weakness. Among the lab results, the nurse notes a WBC count of 2000 and a reversed T-cell/B-cell ratio. This clinical picture is indicative of:
    1. DIC
    2. AIDS
    3. STDs
    4. Anemia

    Answer: 2. AIDS

    Rationale: The signs and symptoms, in addition to a low WBC count, and the reversed T-cell result are among the diagnostic criteria for AIDS.

    Nursing process: Evaluation

    Client need: Physiological integrity

    Clinical skill level: 3

- The AIDS patient is prescribed zidovudine (retrovir or AZT). The patient is told the drug will decrease severity of opportunistic infections related to AIDS. AZT is not considered a cure because it:
    1. Is not strong enough
    2. Is not a broad spectrum drug
    3. Has too many dramatic side effects
    4. Will not kill the AIDS virus

    Answer: 4. Will not kill the AIDS virus

    Rationale: While AZT can decrease the number of HIV in the blood, it cannot eliminate HIV.

    Client need: Physiological integrity

    Nursing process: Intervention

    Clinical skill level: 3

ANAPHYLAXIS

DEFINITION
Anaphylaxis is one of the four principal types of hypersensitivity. Anaphylactoid reactions are a response by the immune system to a known allergen to which the victim has been previously exposed and is highly sensitized.

PATHOPHYSIOLOGY
IgE antibodies are released after exposure to an allergen—such as a drug or an insect bite. Mast cells release histamine and leukotrienes, causing bronchial constriction, angioedema, pruritus, nausea, vomiting and shock. Angioedema is a vascular reaction that involves dilation and increasing permeability of capillaries. This is characterized by localized edema and wheals. The IgE bound mast cells degranulate, releasing mediators which attack organs, cause clinical allergy symptoms, and damage tissue.

ASSOCIATED MEDICAL CONDITIONS
- Allergic asthma
- Angioedema
- Allergic rhinitis
- Anaphylactic shock

NURSING ASSESSMENT
Early onset:
- Localized itching
- Sneezing
- Edema

Within minutes:
- Wheezing
- Cyanosis
- Rapid, weak pulse
- Dilated pupils
- Angioedema
- Dyspnea
- Circulatory shock
- Hypotension
- Bronchial edema

CLIENT NEED
Physiological integrity

NURSING INTERVENTIONS
- Establish airway
- Administer epinephrine SC for laryngeal edema
- Administer diphenhydramine IM or IV; ranitidine, cimetidine
- Remove stinger if present in case of insect bite
- Elevate legs and keep warm
- Apply tourniquet to reduce blood flow from source of antigen
- Administer hydrocortisone IV and repeat epinephrine for extended reactions
- Give fluids, volume expanders, vasosuppressors to maintain blood pressure

PATIENT TEACHING
- Identify and avoid allergen
- If medication has been previously prescribed, take exactly as directed
- Stress management program to control allergic reactions aggravated by stress
- Avoid drugs which produce allergic reactions
- Importance of maintaining an allergy-free environment to control aeroallergens
- Wear medic alert bracelet

ASSOCIATED NURSING DIAGNOSES
- Anxiety
- Fatigue
- Breathing pattern, ineffective
- Powerlessness
- Noncompliance
- Injury, high risk for
- Tissue perfusion, altered: peripheral

STUDY QUESTIONS

■ The nurse is administering penicillin IM to a patient who has never received a penicillin injection. The patient states he is "prone to allergies" but cannot be specific. The patient should be:
1. Given Benadryl po before the injection
2. Tested for allergies ASAP
3. Given epinephrine SC as a prophylactic
4. Closely monitored for at least 20 minutes

Answer: 4. Closely monitored for at least 20 minutes

Rationale: Anytime a new drug or diagnostic medication is injected into a patient, close observation is required to assess an anaphylactic reaction.

Client need: Physiological integrity

Nursing process: Assessment

Clinical skill level: 2

■ The nurse is administering flu shots to elderly patients. It is important to assess each patient for allergy to:
1. Milk
2. Eggs
3. Fish
4. Wheat

Answer: 2. Eggs

Rationale: Influenza immunizations are contraindicated in patients who are allergic to eggs.

Client need: Physiological integrity

Nursing process: Assessment

Clinical skill level: 4

■ The nurse assesses severe dyspnea, tachypnea, and stridor in the patient suffering an anaphylactic reaction. The next complication she should be prepared to intervene in is:
1. DIC
2. Hemorrhage
3. Airway obstruction
4. Cardiac arrest

Answer: 3. Airway obstruction

Rationale: Stridor signals laryngeal edema which, if not controlled through emergency administration of medications, will block the airway.

Client need: Physiological integrity

Nursing process: Evaluation

Clinical skill level: 4

INFECTION

DEFINITION
The invasion of microorganisms that cause the clinical signs and symptoms of illness or a disease process.

PATHOPHYSIOLOGY
The pathophysiology depends upon the type of organism. Basically, there are two types: viral and bacterial. Viral are noncellular organisms that reproduce only within a living cell, and bacteria are organisms that seek a portal into the body.

ASSOCIATED MEDICAL CONDITIONS
- Pneumonia
- Influenza
- Measles
- Respiratory tract infections
- Urinary tract infections
- Nosocomial infections
- Pneumococcal infections
- Tetanus

ASSESSMENT
- Pain
- Chills
- Diaphoresis
- Swelling
- Vital signs q 4°, (especially temperature >101°)
- Any site that may be a portal for entry (wounds, IV)
- Urinary frequency, burning
- Substance abuse
- Fever
- Heat
- Erythema
- Malaise
- WBC and differential
- Culture and sensitivity (before antibiotics started)
- Blood cultures, when indicated

Susceptibility to infection:
Age, diabetes mellitus, other disease processes, steroid therapy, nutritional deficiencies especially protein/Vitamin A and Vitamin C.

CLIENT NEED
Physiological integrity

NURSING INTERVENTIONS
- Universal precautions
- Thoroughly assess patient with history of recent contacts, especially insects, bites, soil
- Use disposable equipment when possible
- Isolate the patient according to CDC guidelines
- Scrupulous handwashing
- Change linens and handle appropriately
- Practice appropriate isolation techniques
- Report disease to state agency or CDC, as required by state law

MEDICAL INTERVENTIONS
- Medications, as appropriate to the specific disease process

PATIENT TEACHING
- Possibility of cross-infection at home
- If susceptibility high, avoid persons with colds, cough
- Need for current immunizations

ASSOCIATED NURSING DIAGNOSES
- Anxiety
- Infection, high risk for (secondary)
- Hyperthermia
- Social isolation
- Body temperature, high risk for
- Fatigue
- Home maintenance management, impaired
- Pain
- Skin integrity, impaired

STUDY QUESTIONS

■ A patient has been diagnosed with meningitis. The nurse institutes which type of isolation?
1. Strict
2. Respiratory
3. Contact
4. Enteric

Answer: 2. Respiratory

Rationale: Respiratory isolation is imposed when a disease is spread by direct or indirect contact or by airborne route.

Client need: Safe effective care environment

Nursing process: Intervention

Clinical skill level: 2

■ (AFB) isolation has been ordered for a recently admitted patient. This isolation is for patients who are diagnosed with:
1. Syphilis
2. Smallpox
3. Tuberculosis
4. Pediculosis

Answer: 3. Tuberculosis

Rationale: The CDC recommends AFB including the use of particle-resistant masks when caring for a TB patient.

Client need: Safe, effective care environment

Nursing process: Intervention

Clinical skill level: 2

■ In instituting Universal precautions, the nurse must approach all patients with the assumption that each patient:
1. Has some kind of infection
2. Must be offered protection
3. Has HIV or HBV infection
4. Has potential for tuberculosis

Answer: 3. Has HIV or HBV infection

Rationale: The CDC recommends, and OSHA requires, Universal precautions because ALL patients must be approached as if they are HIV or HBV positive.

Client need: Safe, effective care environment

Nursing process: Intervention

Clinical skill level: 1

■ The nurse is monitoring a patient with septicemia; signs and symptoms of infection are obvious. What other sign might signal complications in this patient?
1. Fever
2. Diarrhea
3. Hypotension
4. Hypertension

Answer: 2. Hypotension

Rationale: A drop in blood pressure may signal that this patient is going into septic shock.

Client need: Physiological integrity

Nursing process: Evaluation

Clinical skill level: 4

SYSTEMIC LUPUS ERYTHEMOUS (SLE)

DEFINITION
A chronic, inflammatory autoimmune vascular and connective tissue disease that affects every system in the body. Remissions and exacerbations characterize the disorder.

PATHOPHYSIOLOGY
SLE appears to be caused by an immune reaction or defect that causes excessive production of autoantibodies. The antigens and antibodies that are produced cluster into immune complexes localize in small vessels throughout the body causing vasculitis, inflammation and tissue damage. Family studies have shown a genetic link. Some transient, or reversible, forms of SLE are drug-induced.

ASSOCIATED MEDICAL CONDITIONS
- Myocarditis
- Thrombocytopenia
- Meningitis
- Arthritis
- Glomerulonephritis
- Anemia
- Pneumonitis
- Pericarditis
- Scaley, pruritic skin lesions
- Organic brain syndrome
- Raynaud's phenomenon
- Corneal ulcerations
- Bowel infarction

ASSESSMENT
- Butterfly rash across nose and cheeks
- Fatigue
- Stressors, and coping strategies implemented
- Photosensitivity
- Nausea, vomiting
- Loss of appetite
- Fever (may indicate infection), chronic and recurrent
- Petechiae
- Arthritis, swelling of joints, myalgias
- Anemia
- Diarrhea
- Morning stiffness

CLIENT NEED
Physiological integrity

NURSING INTERVENTIONS
- Maintain skin integrity
- Frequent assessments of cardiopulmonary status
- Assist in surgery
- Plasmapheresis, dialysis, and orthopedic therapeutic and palliative management of signs and symptoms as ordered
- Reduce stress
- Provide balanced regimen of activity and rest
- Provide proper nutrition
- Suppression of inflammation, induction of remission and prevention of untoward complications of illness and drug therapy

PATIENT TEACHING
- Teach positive coping strategies in dealing with stress
- Instruct that pregnancy may cause exacerbations
- Teach range of motion of motion to decrease joint stiffness
- Avoid sunlight
- Teach methods of improving appearance with clothing and cosmetics
- Avoid contact with persons who may have contagious infections.
- Instruct regarding side effects of anti inflammatory medication

ASSOCIATED NURSING DIAGNOSES
- Activity intolerance, high risk for
- Knowledge deficit
- Coping, ineffective individual
- Fatigue
- Pain, chronic
- Decreased cardiac output
- Body image disturbance
- Body temperature, high risk for altered
- Diarrhea
- Nutrition: less than body requirements, altered
- Hopelessness
- Skin integrity, impaired
- Infection, high risk for

STUDY QUESTIONS

■ In planning patient teaching for the patient with SLE, the most important aspect the nurse must emphasize is:
1. Compliance with medical regimen
2. Avoid people with infections
3. Report any weight gain immediately
4. Weight-loss diet and exercise

Answer: 1. Compliance with medical regimen

Rationale: The medical regimen consists of adequate rest, medications, and stress management to avoid the exacerbations that are common in this disorder.

Client need: Physiological integrity

Nursing process: Intervention

Clinical skill level: 4

■ In assessing a young woman just diagnosed with SLE, what characteristic observation is the nurse most likely to assess?
1. Butterfly rash over nose
2. Osteoarthritis in the fingers
3. Progressive neurological deficits
4. Orbital edema around eyes

Answer: 1. Butterfly rash over nose

Rationale: This rash is a cardinal sign of the chronic inflammation of the connective tissues. It is one of the diagnostic criteria for SLE.

Client need: Physiological integrity

Nursing process: Intervention

Clinical skill level: 2

UNIT 4
HEMATOLOGIC SYSTEM

- Anemia
- Disseminated Intravascular Coagulopathy (DIC)
- Leukemia
- Pernicious Anemia
- Sickle Cell Anemia

ANEMIA, IRON DEFICIENCY

DEFINITION
A low red blood cell count, usually associated with a low hemoglobin and/or hematocrit reading. The problem is with a low hemoglobin, such that oxygen delivery to tissues is compromised.

PATHOPHYSIOLOGY
Inadequate erythropoiesis, usually caused by nutritional deficiencies, is the primary cause of iron-deficiency anemia. The erythrocytes are characteristically hypochromic and microcytic.

ASSOCIATED MEDICAL CONDITIONS
- Malnutrition
- Alcoholism
- Pregnancy
- Chronic blood loss via menstruation or gastrointestinal losses

ASSESSMENT
- Weakness
- Pallor
- Concave fingernails
- Fatigue
- Dry skin
- Low hemoglobin
- If cardiac workload is increased to compensate:
  - Tachycardia
  - Dyspnea, especially upon exertion
  - Palpitations
  - Syncope
- Smooth, shiny tongue
- Cheilosis (cracks in corners of mouth)

CLIENT NEED
Physiological integrity

NURSING INTERVENTIONS
- Encourage rest
- Gradually increase level of activity
- Prevent injury
- Encourage adequate nutrition

PATIENT TEACHING
- Heme iron is much better absorbed than nonheme iron. Heme iron is found in meat, fish and poultry. Nonheme iron is found in vegetables, fruits, eggs, and grains.
- Foods that are high in iron:
  - Red meats
  - Beans, navy
  - Dried fruits
  - Fish
  - Blackstrap molasses
  - Potatoes
  - Wheat germ
  - Whole grains
- Instruct to take oral iron with food to avoid gastric irritation

ASSOCIATED NURSING DIAGNOSES
- Cardiac output, decreased
- Fatigue
- Nutrition: less than body requirements, altered
- Coping, ineffective individual
- Infection, high risk for
- Injury, at risk for R/T fatigue and weakness

STUDY QUESTIONS

■ Iron dextram (Imferon) IM has been ordered to the patient with iron-deficiency anemia. This medication should be administered:
1. Intramuscularly
2. Subcutaneous
3. Z-track
4. Intravenously

Answer: 3. Z-track

Rationale: The use of Z-track technique will prevent the medications from leaking out of the tissues, decrease reactions and enhance absorption.

Client need: Physiological integrity

Nursing process: Intervention

Clinical skill level: 2

■ The nurse teaches that the best menu choice for the anemic patient is:
1. Beef
2. Fruit
3. Vegetables
4. Red beans

Answer: 1. Beef

Rationale: Red meat is one of the best sources of iron in the diet. One of the causes of iron deficiency is absorption, and iron from red meat is absorbed more thoroughly than from other sources.

Client need: Health promotion and maintenance

Nursing process: Intervention

Clinical skill level: 2

DISSEMINATED INTRAVASCULAR COAGULOPATHY

DEFINITION
Disseminated intravascular coagulopathy is widespread coagulation of the microcirculation throughout the body leading to tissue hypoxia and acidosis.

PATHOPHYSIOLOGY
Causes of DIC include tissue coagulation factors being introduced into the circulation, damage to vascular endothelium, stagnant blood flow, and infection. Widespread clotting in small blood vessels takes place, using up clotting factors and platelets and causing overstimulation of the fibrinolytic system. The bleeding which results from this may range from slight internal bleeding to serious hemorrhaging. Factors which lead to the development of DIC include shock, bacterial and viral infections, tissue damage, retaining a dead fetus in the womb, snake bite and neoplasms.

ASSOCIATED MEDICAL CONDITIONS
- Liver disease
- Septicemia
- Toxemia of pregnancy
- Biliary obstruction
- Multi-trauma
- Vitamin K deficiency (Hypothrombinemia)

ASSESSMENT
- Spontaneous bleeding from all body orifices
- Spontaneous bleeding from IV, IM sites
- Purpura
- Tachycardia
- Oliguria
- Prolonged prothrombin time (PT)
- Ecchymoses
- Spontaneous bleeding from gums
- Petechiae (especially at pressure sites)
- Hematuria
- Diaphoresis
- Lack of clotting
- Increased partial thromboplastin time (PPT)
- Acral cyanosis

CLIENT NEED
Physiological integrity

NURSING INTERVENTIONS
- Fluid replacement
- RBCs
- Cryoprecipitate (low fibrinogen level)
- Monitor/assess renal function
- Correct cause or underlying condition
- Administer intravenous heparin to decrease hemorrhaging and hinder coagulation
- Fresh frozen plasma
- Platelets
- IV Heparin (to promote coagulation)
- Assess for occult and overt bleeding
- Monitor fluid volume/coagulation factor replacement
- Cryoprecipitate or fresh frozen plasma-to replace clotting factors

ASSOCIATED NURSING DIAGNOSES
- Anxiety
- Injury, at high risk for
- Fluid volume deficit, high risk for
- Ventilation, inability to sustain spontaneous
- Fear
- Knowledge deficit
- Spiritual distress (distress of the human spirit)
- Tissue perfusion, altered (peripheral)

STUDY QUESTIONS

■ In monitoring the patient with DIC, what is the most common complication that is likely to occur?
1. Shock
2. Cardiac arrest
3. Renal failure
4. Liver failure

Answer: 1. Shock

Rationale: Because of the tendency toward bleeding, shock is always a threat in DIC.

Client need: Physiological Integrity

Nursing process: Asesessment

Clinical skill level: 3

■ The patient in critical condition with DIC must be closely observed for :
1. Myocardial infarction
2. Septic shock
3. Pneumonia
4. Pulmonary embolism

Answer: 4. Pulmonary embolism

Rationale: A cardinal clinical finding in DIC is the hemorrhaging and thrombus formation that occurs simultaneously. A thrombus that could break away and become an emboli is the threat.

Client need: Physiological integrity

Nursing process: Assessment

Clinical skill level: 4

■ Heparin is being administered to the patient with DIC. The nurse is aware that heparin therapy is difficult to control in this patient because DIC:
1. PTT is already prolonged
2. Clotting time is decreased
3. RBCs are quickly destroyed
4. Platelets deteriorate

Answer: 1. PTT is already prolonged

Rationale: Heparin is given to interfere with intravascular clotting. However, since thrombus formation is concurrent with bleeding, heparin treatment involves a risk.

Client need: Physiological integrity

Nursing process: Evaluation

Clinical skill level: 4

LEUKEMIA

DEFINITION
Leukemia is a neoplastic disorder of the blood-forming tissue, and primarily targets the spleen, lymph nodes, and bone marrow.

PATHOPHYSIOLOGY
This disease is characterized by the abnormally uncontrolled growth of immature leukocytes. The white cells most affected are the lymphocytes, granulocytes, and monocytes. The immaturity of the white cells leads to decreased immunocompetence with increased susceptibility to infection.

ASSOCIATED MEDICAL CONDITIONS
- Acute Granulocytic Leukemia (AGL)
- Acute Lymphocytic Leukemia (ALL)
- Chronic Granulocytic Leukemia (CGL)
- Chronic Lymphocytic Leukemia (CLL)

ASSESSMENT
- Fatigue
- Chronic malaise
- Dizziness
- Nosebleeds
- Petechiae
- Weight loss
- Sensitivity/pain in mid-sternal area, deep bone pain
- Hepato/Splenomegaly
- Anemia
- Pallor
- Fever (without infection)
- Bleeding gums
- Ecchymoses (easily bruised)
- Anorexia
- Marked increase in immature leukocytes
- Frequent infections

CLIENT NEED
Physiological integrity

NURSING INTERVENTIONS
- Provide adequate rest
- Protect from falls, trauma
- Protective isolation
- Administer blood/blood products
- Provide appropriate oral hygiene
- Force fluids, 3-4 liter/day
- Constant monitoring for bleeding/hemorrhage
- Administer stool softeners
- Supportive therapy to patient/family

MEDICAL INTERVENTIONS
- Bone marrow biopsy
- Bone marrow transplant
- Chemotherapy

PATIENT TEACHING
- Avoid exertion
- Avoid people with colds/infections
- Protect against injury
- Teach adequate nutritional intake; high calorie, high protein

NURSING DIAGNOSES
- Anxiety
- Fear
- Body temperature, high risk for altered
- Pain
- Powerlessness
- Skin integrity, high risk for impaired
- Infection, at high risk for
- Body image disturbance
- Fatigue
- Nutrition: less than body requirements, altered
- Physical mobility, impaired
- Depression
- Spiritual distress (distress of the human spirit)

STUDY QUESTIONS

■ Teaching for the patient undergoing a bone marrow aspiration should include diaphramatic breathing and relaxation techniques because:
1. The procedure is tedious
2. Pain is tense for several days
3. Aspiration causes pain
4. Complications can be expected

Answer: 3. Aspiration causes pain

Rationale: The patient should be instructed that there will be pain upon aspiration and how to cope with this discomfort. The site may ache for two or three days after procedure.

Nursing process: Intervention

Client need: Health promotion and maintenance

Clinical skill level: 2

■ The patient's platelet count is assessed prior to bone marrow aspiration because:
1. Platelets are lost in aspiration
2. It indicates presence of infection
3. Blood may be too thick to aspirate
4. Hemorrhage is a risk

Answer: 4. Hemorrhage is a risk

Rationale: The hazard of hemorrhage is increased if the platelet count is low.

Nursing process: Assessment

Client need: Physiological integrity

Clinical skill level: 3

- Following the bone marrow aspiration procedure, the nurse applies a pressure dressing and asks the patient to:
    1. Assume a sitting position
    2. Lie in a recumbent position
    3. Lie in a prone position
    4. Turn and cough periodically

    Answer: 2. Lie in a recumbent position

    Rationale: The recumbent position will apply additional pressure to the aspiration site to prevent the risk of hemorrhage

    Nursing process: Intervention

    Client need: Physiological integrity

    Clinical skill level: 2

- The treatment plan for the leukemia patient reads: force fluids, 150 cc per hour. The rationale for forcing fluids is to:
    1. Prevent need for IVs
    2. Enhance urinary output
    3. Provide adequate calories
    4. Prevent dehydration

    Answer: 4. Prevent dehydration

    Rationale: This patient is at risk for dehydration as body fluids are depleted due to fever and anorexia.

    Nursing process: Intervention

    Client need: Physiological integrity

    Clinical skill level: 2

■ Which medication is prescribed to inhibit the formation of uric acid crystals in the leukemia patient?
1. Zovirax
2. Zorprin
3. Allopurinol
4. Azotrex

Answer: 3. Allopurinol

Rationale: Leukemia patients have high levels of uric acid resulting from the massive destruction of leukocytes by the chemotherapy.

Nursing process: Intervention

Client need: Physiological integrity

Clinical skill level: 4

■ The physician diagnoses leukemia. What would the laboratory report indicate?
1. Large numbers of immature WBCs
2. Large numbers of RBCs and platelets
3. Large numbers of mature white blood cells
4. A radical change in plasma neutrophils

Answer: 1. Large numbers of immature WBCs

Rationale: The hallmark of leukemia is fast multiplication of young, immature white blood cells referred to as blasts.

Nursing process: Assessment

Client need: Physiological integrity

Clinical skill level: 2

PERNICIOUS ANEMIA

DEFINITION
This disorder results from a deficiency of Vitamin B_{12}, specifically the intrinsic factor. It is a chronic, progressive megaloblastic anemia, which is fatal if untreated.

PATHOPHYSIOLOGY
The deficiency of Vitamin B_{12} occurs when there is a lack of intrinsic factor — a protein substance required for the absorption of Vitamin B_{12} in the small intestine. The myelin matter of the dorsal and lateral columns of the spine is affected.

ASSOCIATED MEDICAL CONDITIONS
- Hyperthyroidism
- Celiac disease
- Total gastrectomy
- Tape worm infestation

ASSESSMENT
- Beefy, red tongue
- Anorexia
- Tinnitus
- Diarrhea
- Shortness of breath
- Mood swings
- Numbness, tingling in extremities
- Enlarged spleen
- Constipation
- Weakness
- Indigestion
- Weight loss
- Dizziness
- Palpitation with angina
- Early gray hair
- Lemon-yellow tint in skin color
- Tachycardia

CLIENT NEED
Physiological integrity

NURSING INTERVENTIONS
- Treat symptoms
- Provide adequate rest
- Promote adequate nutritional intake
- Administer B_{12} injections
- Provide frequent oral hygiene
- Monitor neurological symptoms

MEDICAL INTERVENTIONS
- Order Schilling Test
- Gastrectomy

PATIENT TEACHING
- Teach that B_{12} therapy will be necessary for lifetime, usually twice a month
- Avoid foods that are spicy or difficult to digest
- Stress necessity of blood exams and examination of fecal matter every six months.

STUDY QUESTIONS

■ Pernicious anemia is a disorder in the older patient that is caused by the lack of an intrinsic factor that interferes with absorption of a substance. What is that substance?
 1. Folic acid
 2. Ferrous sulfate
 3. Vitamin B_{12}
 4. Vitamin K

Answer: 3. Vitamin B_{12}

Rationale: Intrinsic factor is the protein substance essential for Vitamin B_{12} to be absorbed in the small intestine.

Nursing process: Assessment

Client need: Physiological integrity

Clinical skill level: 2

- What does a Schilling Test measure?
    1. Spleen enlargement
    2. Thrombocytopenia
    3. B$_{12}$ absorption
    4. Gastric juice analysis

    Answer: 3. B$_{12}$ absorption

    Rationale: The Schilling test for B$_{12}$ absorption, especially if any other signs of pernicious anemia are noted.

    Client need: Physiological integrity

    Nursing process: Evaluation

    Clinical skill level: 4

- What is a classic sign of pernicious anemia?
    1. Indigestion
    2. Diarrhea
    3. Red, beefy tongue
    4. Flushed appeareance

    Answer: 3. Red beefy tongue

    Rationale: The non-absorption of Vitamin B$_{12}$ and the intrinsic factor causes several signs and symptoms, the cardinal sign being the smooth, red, enlarged tongue.

    Client need: Physiological integrity

    Nursing process: Assessment

    Clinical skill level: 3

- The patient diagnosed with pernicious anemia will require B_{12} injections:
    1. For a week
    2. For 10 days
    3. For 3 months
    4. For life

    Answer: 3. For life

    Rationale: The B_{12} deficiency, along with a deficiency in the intrinsic factor, is a life-long problem that is not cured but is controlled with injections.

    Client need: Physiological integrity

    Nursing process: Assessment

    Clinical skill level: 3

- How should HCL be administered to the patient with pernicious anemia?
    1. IM
    2. PO
    3. Sublingual
    4. Through a straw

    Answer: 4. Through a straw

    Rationale: HCL will stain the teeth and should be administered through a straw after meals even after it is diluted.

    Client need: Physiological integrity

    Nursing process: Intervention

    Clinical skill level: 3

SICKLE CELL ANEMIA

DEFINITION
A genetic disorder (homozygous) in which a person has two HbS hemoglobin genes instead of HbA hemoglobin genes.

PATHOPHYSIOLOGY
The Hbs hemoglobin forms crystalloid molecules in the RBCs when the oxygen supply to these cells is limited. The molecules cause the RBCs to become sickle-shaped and to die quickly. Blood circulation slows, leading to hypoxia and further sickling. The sickled cells clump together and clog small blood vessels leading to decreased tissue perfusion, hypoxia, organ infarction and necrosis.

MOST COMMON MEDICAL CONDITIONS
- Sickle cell disease
- Sickle trait
- Sickle thalassemia

ASSESSMENT
- Dyspnea with exertion
- Pallor
- Gallstones may develop
- Enlargement of the frontal skull
- Seizures
- Leg ulcers
- Jaundice
- Brownish-orange urine
- Fever
- Excruciating pain (especially during crisis) of joints
- Limitation of mobility
- Tachycardia

CLIENT NEED
Physiological integrity

NURSING INTERVENTIONS
- Prevent dehydration
- Administer O$_2$
- Strict isolation to protect from infections
- Administer pain medications
- Keep warm
- Administer IV fluids
- Administer folic acid to prevent depletion

MEDICAL INTERVENTIONS
- Hemoglobin electrophoresis to diagnose disease
- Infusion of hypotonic solutions to enlarge RBCs
- Tranfusions with packed RBCs if the hemoglobin falls below 7 to 10 g/d.

PATIENT TEACHING
- Seek genetic counseling
- Maintain adequate nutrition/hydration
- Avoid smoking
- Avoid exposure to cold
- Avoid activities which will result in limited oxygen supply

ASSOCIATED NURSING DIAGNOSES
- Activity intolerance, high risk for
- Body temperature, high risk for altered
- Anxiety
- Fear
- Hopelessness
- Hypothermia
- Parenting, high risk for altered
- Caregiver role strain, high risk for
- Breathing pattern, ineffective
- Fatigue
- Fluid volume deficit, high risk for
- Hyperthermia
- Injury, high risk for
- Tissue perfusion, altered: peripheral

STUDY QUESTIONS

■ What is the primary cause of a sickle cell crisis?
1. Sickled blood cells lodged in small vessels
2. Viscosity of the blood thickens
3. Thickened blood causes obstructions
4. Cells in marrow cause bone pain

Answer: 1. Sickled blood cells lodged in small vessels
Rationale: During a sickle cell crisis, oxygen to red blood cells becomes limited, causing the hemoglobin to crystalize in the cell. This causes the cells to alter in shaping, becoming sickled and sticky. The sickle cells die in 7-10 days, clumps together, and clog blood vessels.
Nursing process: Evaluation
Client need: Physiological integrity

Clinical skill level: 3

■ Family planning is essential in patient teaching regarding sickle cell anemia because this disorder is:
1. Communicable
2. Genetic
3. Contagious
4. Infectious

Answer: 2. Genetic
Rationale: Sickle cell anemia occurs in blacks and persons of mediterranean descent who have two HbS hemoglobin genes rather than the normal HbA hemoglobin genes. Persons with this should be counseled that ¼ of their children will have the disease, ½ will have the sickle cell trait, and ¼ will have the normal gene.
Nursing process: Evaluation
Client need: Physiological integrity

Clinical skill level: 1

■ Sickle cell crisis results primarily in situations when there is an inadequate amount of what substance?
1. Iron
2. Oxygen
3. Hemoglobin
4. Red blood cells

Answer: 2. Oxygen

Rationale: As the cells sickle, they slow circulation, further reducing oxygen to the surrounding cells and increasing the sickling. The hemoglobin in the sickled cell releases oxygen more easily than does a normal cell.

Nursing process: Assessment

Client need: Physiological integrity

Clinical skill level: 2

■ In planning care for the patient with decreased platelets what precautions should be taken?
1. Do not take the blood pressure
2. Do not take rectal temperature
3. Do not give subcutaneous injections
4. Do not pump cuff 10 points above previous reading

Answer: 4. Do not pump cuff 10 points above previous reading

Rationale: Pumping up the pressure cuff may cause extensive bruising of the arm.

Nursing process: Intervention

Client need: Physiological integrity

Clinical skill level: 2

■ A patient is having a hemolytic reaction to blood. The nurse stops the blood, takes vital signs, and calls the doctor. What other action is important?
1. Save the first voided urine
2. Take blood sample
3. Prepare to restart blood
4. Start solution of D5W

Answer: 2. Take blood sample

Rationale: The lab will need a blood sample to double check the type and crossmatch, and to test for bacterial contamination.

Nursing process: Intervention

Client need: Physiological integrity

> Clinical skill level: 2

■ The patient who is receiving a unit of RBCs begins, rather suddenly, to complain of severe back pain. Routinely the nurse takes vital signs and finds he is hypotensive. This assessment is evaluated as:
1. Normal findings in RBC transfusion
2. Nothing unusual for this patient
3. Transfusion reaction
4. A need to reposition

Answer: 3. Transfusion reaction

Rationale: When the antigen-antibody reaction that occur during a transfusion reaction begin to happen, back pain occurs as a result of the kidney injury that is taking place.

Nursing process: Evaluation

Client need: Physiological integrity

> Clinical skill level: 3

■ The clinical symptoms of polycythemia vera are pruritus, ruddy complexion, dizziness, headache, and angina. These symptoms are:
1. Increased blood viscosity and volume
2. Insidious blood loss
3. Iron deficiency anemia
4. Hemoglobin concentrations

Answer: 1. Increased blood viscosity and volume

Rationale: The marrow cells, for some unexplained reason, escape normal functioning and overproduce. In polycythemia vera the RBC, WBC, and platelet counts are elevated.

Nursing process: Evaluation

Client need: Physiological integrity

Clinical skill level: 2

UNIT 5
NERVOUS SYSTEM

- Alzheimer's Disease
- Cerebrovascular Accident
- Head Injury
- Myasthenia Gravis
- Parkinson's Disease

ALZHEIMER'S DISEASE

DEFINITION
Alzheimer's is an organic brain syndrome in which the individual suffers a dementia that is characterized by a progressive deterioration in intellect and behavior. The patient experiences loss of memory and changes in personality and judgment. Eventually, he or she is unable to perform activities of daily living.

PATHOPHYSIOLOGY
A relationship between Alzheimer's and the trisomy 21 Down's syndrome is being studied. A chromosome 21 defect has been discovered in Alzheimer's patients. Damage to neurons occurs in the brain, particularly in the cerebral cortex. Cells that are most affected utilize the neurotransmitter, acetylcholine. Since acetylcholine is instrumental in memory, the signs of Alzheimer's are directly linked to this problem.

ASSOCIATED MEDICAL CONDITIONS
- Degenerative dementia
- Organic brain syndrome
- Delirium

ASSESSMENT
Early stages:
- Recent memory loss (remote memory stays intact)
- Increasing irritability
- Apathy toward important issues
- Decline in cognitive functioning:
  - Problem-solving
  - Decision making
  - Critical judgment
  - Abstract thinking
  - Lack of ability to handle business and/or personal affairs

As disease progresses:
- Disorientation
- Wandering around; getting lost
- Perseveration (repeats words, phrases)
- Depression (because patient is aware of what is happening)
- Confabulation (recreating events)
- Increasingly restless
- Talks to self
- Urinary, fecal incontinence
- Emotional lability
- Anomia (cannot name things)
- Circumlocution (talks in circles)
- Loss of insight or memory (Does not know what to do ever regarding simple tasks)
- Appearance of primitive reflexes
- Cogwheel rigidity
- Inappropriate chewing

In final stage of disease:
- No communication
- Seizures
- Immobility
- Contractures
- Masked affect
- Delusions
- Fetal position
- Refuses to eat

CLIENT NEED
Safe effective care, environment

NURSING INTERVENTIONS
- Administer tricyclic antidepressant for depression
- Administer Valium or Librium for anxiety and agitation
- Provide for safety
- Administer mild sedatives for sleep (Benadryl or chloral hydrate)
- Administer major tranquilizer (such as Thorazine) for increasing agitation

PATIENT TEACHING

- Explain potential miscommunication, particularly confabulation
- Explain safety requirements
- Importance of keeping identification tag on patient at all times
- Warn that the patient is prone to wander around, unlock doors, and get lost
- Explain that the patient may be incapable of simple tasks

ASSOCIATED NURSING DIAGNOSES

- Activity intolerance
- Anxiety
- Caregiver role strain, high risk for
- Injury, high risk for
- Fatigue
- Hopelessness
- Family coping, disabling, ineffective
- Protection, altered
- Personal identity disturbance
- Social isolation
- Thought process, altered
- Adjustment, impaired
- Body image disturbance
- Communication, impaired verbal
- Family processes, altered
- Fear
- Incontinence, total
- Nutrition: less than body requirements, altered
- Powerlessness
- Sensory/perceptual alterations: kinesthetic, tactile
- Sleep pattern disturbance

STUDY QUESTIONS

■ In teaching the family care of the Alzheimer's patient, the nurse emphasizes which of the following behaviors as a serious threat to safety:
1. Circumlocution
2. Perseveration
3. Emotional lability
4. Wandering around

Answer: 4. Wandering around

Rationale: The Alzheimer's patient tends to wander around and, unable to focus on cognitive problem-solving abilities, usually gets lost.

Nursing Process: Intervention

Client Need: Physiological integrity

> Clinical skill level: 2

■ The nurse prepares to administer a mild sedative to the restless Alzheimer's patient. Which of the following is most likely to be prescribed?
1. Benadryl
2. Secobarbital
3. Pentobarbital
4. Methabarbital

Answer: 1. Benadryl

Rationale: Barbiturates should be avoided because they depress CNS function and could cause confusion, especially in the patient with dementia.

Nursing Process: Intervention

Client Need: Physiological integrity

> Clinical skill level: 3

■ A patient has been recently diagnosed with Alzheimer's disease. When teaching the family about the prognosis, the nurse must explain that:
1. It progresses gradually with deterioration of functions
2. Many individuals can be cured if diagnosis is made early
3. Diet and exercise can slow the process considerably
4. Few patients live for more than 3 years after diagnosis

Answer: 1. It progresses gradually with deterioration of functions

Rationale: Alzheimer's disease is degenerative and is not curable. A progressive loss of neurologic functioning is the major clinical manifestation of this disease, and therefore, is the priority clinical factor.

Nursing process: Intervention

Client need: Health promotion and maintenance

Clinical skill level: 2

■ When the elderly Alzheimer's patient becomes agitated and disoriented, which medication is most likely to be prescribed?
1. Thorazine
2. Haldol
3. Melleril
4. Elavil

Answer: 2. Haldol

Rationale: This antipsychotic medication has proven to be the most effective in decreasing the restlessness and agitation of Alzheimer's patients.

Client need: Physiological integrity

Nursing process: Intervention

Clinical skill level: 2

CEREBROVASCULAR ACCIDENT

DEFINITION
A CVA is an infarction that occurs in the brain. It is usually caused by a thrombus, an embolism, or hemorrhage.

PATHOPHYSIOLOGY
Cerebral infarction occurs when a local area of the brain is deprived of blood. Local or general disorders may cause the alteration of the blood supply. If cerebral circulation is interrupted extensively, cerebral anoxia, or lack of oxygen to the brain, develops. After 10 minutes, changes to the brain resulting from cerebral anoxia are irreversible.

ASSOCIATED MEDICAL CONDITIONS
- Cerebral embolism
- Vascular malformation
- Intracranial bleeding
- Cerebral thrombosis
- Subarachnoid hemorrhage
- Intracerebral hemorrhage

ASSESSMENT
- Pupil response
- Rhythm and depth of respirations
- Level of consciousness
- Decerebrate posturing
- Decorticate posturing

CLIENT NEED
Physiological integrity

NURSING INTERVENTIONS
- Maintain airway
- Suction prn
- Foley catheter
- Watch for thrombophlebitis
- Keep patient turned to side
- Monitor I&O
- Monitor LOC
- Auscultate breath sounds (pneumonia a threat)

MEDICAL INTERVENTIONS
- Arteriography
- MRI
- CT scan

PATIENT TEACHING
- Self-care
- Bladder-retraining for incontinence
- Importance of self-sufficiency
- Continue exercising
- Retraining in sitting, standing, ambulation
- Take coumadin exactly as prescribed

ASSOCIATED NURSING DIAGNOSES
- Activity intolerance, high risk for
- Body image disturbance
- Anxiety
- Hopelessness
- Injury, high risk for
- Sensory/perceptual alterations: visual, auditory, kinesthetic, gustatory
- Nutrition, less than body requirements, altered
- Caregiver role strain, high risk for
- Communication, impaired verbal
- Fear
- Incontinence, total
- Unilateral neglect
- Self-care deficit: bathing/hygiene, dressing/grooming, feeding, toileting
- Peripheral neurovascular dysfunction, high risk for

STUDY QUESTIONS

■ When the nurse is assisting a patient with hemiplegia or hemiparesis in walking, the nurse should always:
1. Stand at the unaffected side
2. Stand behind the patient
3. Place patient in a wheel chair
4. Stand at the affected side

Answer: 4. Stand at the affected side

Rationale: Hemiplegia or hemiparesis is the dysfunction, or weakness, of one side of the body due to an injury to the motor areas of the brain. Therefore, the patient may need assistance in utilizing the affected side.

Nursing process: Intervention

Client need: Safe, effective care environment

Clinical skill level: 2

■ The nurse assesses a patient experiencing global aphasia. She realizes that this patient:
1. Cannot recognize people
2. Cannot write
3. Cannot express feelings
4. Cannot talk

Answer: 4. Cannot talk

Rationale: Global aphasia is injury or disease to the brain centers that results in the disturbance of both verbal and perceptive language functioning.

Nursing process: Assessment

Client need: Physiological integrity

Clinical skill level: 2

■ What is the most life-threatening complication the nurse must be alert for in caring for the patient with a CVA?
1. Hypertension
2. Hypotension
3. Oligura
4. Increasing intracranial pressure

Answer: 4. Increasing intracranial pressure
Rationale: In a CVA a cerebral hemorrhage can increase intracranial volume, causing IICP. If not monitored and treated promptly, brain herniation and death will occur.
Nursing process: Assessment
Client need: Physiological integrity

Clinical skill level: 3

■ What critical intervention must the nurse perform in a CVA emergency?
1. Without tilting the neck, elevate the head
2. Tilting the head forward, elevate the head
3. Tilting the neck backwards, elevate the head
4. Avoid moving the head, keeping it flat

Answer: 1. Without tilting the neck, elevate the head.
Rationale: The head must be slightly elevated about 30 degrees to enhance venous return and prevent aspiration. The neck should not be flexed because compression of the jugular veins may cause IICP.
Nursing process: Intervention
Client need: Physiological integrity

Clinical skill level: 3

■ A stroke patient has absence of the blink reflex on the affected side. Which intervention is a priority when planning nursing care?
1. Place an eye pad over affected eye
2. Apply an eye shield to affected eye
3. Instill artificial tears to both eyes
4. Instill normal saline in both eyes

Answer: 2. Apply an eye shield to affected eye

Rationale: An eye shield will prevent the eye from drying. It also eliminates the second image and provides clear vision from the unaffected eye.

Nursing process: Intervention

Client need: Physiological integrity

Clinical skill level: 2

■ When increasing intracranial pressure is suspected, the nurse should be alert for what other signs and symptoms?
1. Confusion and paranoia
2. Blindness and tinnitus
3. Headaches and delusions
4. Projectile vomiting and headaches

Answer: 4. Projectile vomiting and headaches

Rationale: As IICP increases, swelling tissues exert pressure on cerebral blood vessels, the dura mater and other structures in the brain and back of the eye.

Nursing process: Evaluation

Client need: Physiological integrity

Clinical skill level: 2

■ The nurse is assessing a patient for a cerebrovascular accident. Which symptoms does the patient describe he experienced just before the stroke occurred?
1. Palpitations
2. Disorientation
3. Vertigo or dizziness
4. Euphoria

Answer: 3. Vertigo or dizziness

Rationale: A CVA occurs when part of the brain dies because the blood supply to that area of the brain is insufficient. This lack of circulation causes dizziness and vertigo.

Nursing process:

Client need:

Clinical skill level: 3

■ A cerebrovascular accident has left the patient with homonymous hemianopsia, blindness in half of his visual field. This symptom manifests itself in what way?
1. Increased preference for sweets
2. Eating food on only half the plate
3. Forgetting the names of friends
4. Inability to chew and swallow

Answer: 2. Eating food on only half the plate

Rationale: Because the patient is not able to see the food on the other half of the plate—the half on his affected side—he treats the food as though it does not exist.

Nursing process: Evaluation

Client need: Physiological integrity

Clinical skill level: 2

■ The physican restricts IV fluids and orders diuretics for a CVA patient. The rationale for this is:
  1. To increase cardiac output
  2. To minimize incontinence
  3. To reduce cerebral edema
  4. To reduce threat of embolism

  Answer: 3. To reduce cerebral edema
  Rationale: The physician is attempting to decrease circulating volume and thereby decrease cerebral edema.
  Nursing process: Evaluation
  Client need: Physiological integrity

  > Clinical skill level: 3

■ The patient's prothrombin time indicates that the patient has not been taking Coumadin regularly. In teaching the patient about the medication, the patient remarks, "I just forget to take it sometimes." The nurse teaches the patient:
  1. To double up on doses when he forgets
  2. Suggest a regimen to keep him on schedule
  3. He can take the drug when he thinks about it
  4. Take the medication every other day if necessary

  Answer: 2. Suggest a regimen to keep him on schedule.
  Rationale: Coumadin must be taken as prescribed in order to maintain the therapeutic range of 20-30 percent normal prothrombin activity. Regular bloodwork must be done to monitor for this range.
  Client need: Physiological integrity
  Nursing process: Intervention

  > Clinical skill level: 2

HEAD INJURY

DEFINITION
A physical impact to the head that causes injury. Head injuries are classified as:
- Concussion
  - Transient interruption of CNS function due to trauma. No cerebral structure damage.
- Contusion:
  - Bruising tissue—may see signs of coup and countercoup
- Coup:
  - Obvious bruising at the injury site
- Countercoup:
  - Bruising, and often, lacerations on the opposite side of the brain that actually sustained the injury.

PATHOPHYSIOLOGY
Head injuries include scalp, skull or brain injuries, usually stemming from an impact. Because the head is a vascular, scalp injuries, which involve lacerations, contusions or abrasions, may result in profuse bleeding. Skull injuries, which include linear, depressed and basiliar skull fractures, are the result of a blow of enough force to injure the brain. Depressed fract ures bruise the brain or drive bone fragments into it. Brain injuries may be open—those that penetrate the skull—or closed.

ASSOCIATED MEDICAL CONDITIONS
- Shock
- Brain stem injury
- Cervical fracure
- Impaired respiration
- Skull fracture
- Epidural and subdural hemorrhage

ASSESSMENT
- Pupils small, equal, reactive
- Hearing loss from auditory nerve damage
- Reaction to stimuli
- Facial paresis or paralysis from facial nerve damage
- Loss of sense of smell from olfactory nerve damage
- Response to command

CLIENT NEED
Physiological integrity

NURSING INTERVENTIONS
- Carefully monitor respirations
- Monitor ECG
- Be alert for SOB
- Administer osmotic diuretics (Mannitol)
- Administer steroids
- Strictly monitor I&O
- Observe color, temperature, pulse
- Support head; do not move neck
- Administer O_2
- Observe color, temperature, pulse
- Strictly monitor IV fluids
- Apply cervical collar

MEDICAL INTERVENTIONS
- Acetaminophen or codeine
- Histamine antagonists, such as cimetidine (Tagamet)
- Antiseizure medications, such as phenytoin

PATIENT TEACHING
- Patient should continue rehabilitation program after going home
- Patient may be given anticonvulsants for 1 to 2 years after injury to control seizures
- Recovery may continue for up to 3 years after injury

ASSOCIATED NURSING DIAGNOSES
- Tissue perfusion, altered: cerebral
- Communication, impaired verbal
- Fear
- Hopelessness
- Pain
- Anxiety
- Sensory/perceptual alterations: visual, tactile
- Body temperature, high risk for altered
- Coping, ineffective individual
- Gas exchange, impaired
- Injury, high risk for
- Self-care deficit
- Swallowing, Impaired

STUDY QUESTIONS

The finding of unequal pupillary response in an unconscious person should alert the nurse to:
1. Poisoning
2. Shock
3. Head injury
4. Overdose

Answer: 3. Head injury

Rationale: Unequal pupils in this patient may indicate that the oculomotor nerve (cranial nerve III) is being compressed by increasing intracranial pressure.

Nursing process: Assessment

Client need: Physiological integrity

Clinical skill level: 3

■ A young man is in the emergency room with a closed head injury following a car accident. Baseline vital signs are BP 120/80, P 78, R 20. Which nursing assessment data would indicate a deterioration in his condition?
1. Vital signs of 110/80, 72, 20
2. Vital signs of 100/60, 70, 30
3. Vital signs of 130/90, 88, 30
4. Vital signs of 160/90, 64, 12

Answer: 4. Vital signs of 160/90, 64, 12

Rationale: Signs of increasing intracranial pressure (IICP) are increasing blood pressure (especially systolic), decreasing pulse, decreasing respirations, and widened pulse pressure.

Nursing process: Assessment

Client need: Physiological integrity

Clinical skill level: 3

- An IV is started on a patient who is suffering a head injury from a car wreck two hours ago. The patient is exhibiting signs suffered of IICP. The nurse will set the fluid rate at:
    1. 30 cc/hr
    2. 75 cc/hr
    3. 100 cc/hr
    4. 125 cc/hr

    Answer: 1. 30 cc/hr

    Rationale: The IV should run at a rate to keep vein open (KVO), which is about 30 cc/hr. Increasing the IV rate would increase circulating volume, thus increasing intracranial pressure.

    Nursing process: Intervention

    Client need: Physiological integrity

    Clinical skill level: 3

- A young man is in the emergency room with a closed head injury. Baseline vital signs are BP 120/80, P 78, R 20. Which nursing assessment data would include a deterioration in his condition?
    1. Vital signs of 110/80, 72, 20
    2. Vital signs of 100/60, 70, 30
    3. Vital signs of 130/90, 88, 30
    4. Vital signs of 160/100, 64, 12

    Answer: 4. Vital signs of 160/100, 64, 12

    Rationale: Signs of increased intracranial pressure are: increasing blood pressure, decreasing pulse, decreasing respirations.

    Client need: Physiological integrity

    Nursing process: Evaluation

    Clinical skill level: 4

MYASTHENIA GRAVIS

DEFINITION
A neuromuscular disease characterized by weakness and fatigue.

PATHOPHYSIOLOGY
Myasthenia gravis occurs when antibodies attack the acetylcholine receptor and interfere with neuromuscular transmission.

ASSOCIATED MEDICAL CONDITIONS
- Diplopia
- Dysphonia
- Cholinergic crisis
- Ptosis
- Myasthenia crisis

ASSESSMENT
- Weakness
- Respiratory infection (with aggravate condition)
- Fatigue
- Thyroid dysfunction

CLIENT NEED
Physiological integrity

NURSING INTERVENTIONS
- Monitor breath sounds
- Monitor of aspiration of food/fluids
- Turn, cough, deep breathe to prevent hypostatic pneumonia
- Suction prn
- Recommend structural activities with rest periods
- Bowel-bladder training, if incontinence occurs

MEDICAL INTERVENTIONS
- Prescribe neostigmine
- Low-dose steroids

PATIENT TEACHING
- Avoid conditions which may lead to myasthenic crisis, i.e. emotional upset, infections, exposure to heat and cold, and physical exertion.
- Encourage to utilize self-help or adaptive devices.

ASSOCIATED NURSING DIAGNOSES
- Activity intolerance, high risk for
- Anxiety
- Infection, high risk for
- Home maintenance management, impaired
- Coping, ineffective individual
- Fatigue
- Hopelessness

STUDY QUESTIONS

■ A 28-year-old woman complains of extreme muscle weakness and states, "I have to rest even after talking for a little while." The nurse assesses her for other symptoms of:
1. Multiple sclerosis
2. Hepatitis B
3. Thyroid disorder
4. Myasthenia gravis

Answer: 4. Myasthenia gravis

Rationale: Myasthenia gravis, a disease that causes weakness in voluntary muscles, is most common in women, age 20-30.

Client need: Physiological integrity

Nursing process: Assessment

Clinical skill level: 3

- Other early symptoms of myasthenia gravis that the nurse assesses are:
    1. Urinary and fecal incontinence
    2. Nausea and vomiting
    3. Diplopia and ptosis
    4. Abdominal cramping and diarrhea

    Answer: 3. Diplopia and ptosis

    Rationale: Because of the involvement of the ocular muscles this patient often exhibits a "mask" or sleepy expression.

    Client need: Physiological integrity

    Nursing process: Assessment

    Clinical skill level: 4

- The nurse is planning patient teaching for this recently-diagnosed patient. What is the drug most often prescribed in myasthenia gravis?
    1. Valium
    2. Tennuate
    3. Tensilon
    4. Mestinon

    Answer: 4. Mestinon

    Rationale: Pyridostigmine bromide (mestinon) allows acetylcholine to accumulate, stimulating the receptors of the muscles. Tensilon is used as a diagnostic acid only.

    Client need: Physiological integrity

    Nursing process: Intervention

    Clinical skill level: 3

- A priority of nursing care that must be emphasized to the patient with myasthenia gravis is:
    1. Encourage active ROM exercises
    2. Recommend enemas for constipation
    3. Give medications exactly as ordered
    4. Exercise regime to build muscle strength

    Answer: 3. Give medications exactly as ordered

    Rationale: If medication is not given on schedule, the muscles may relax and the patient may lose the ability to swallow.

    Client need: Physiological integrity

    Nursing process: Intervention

    Clinical skill level: 3

- The nurse is aware that the ultimate danger in this disease is progressive weakness and, eventually, the onset of myasthenic crisis. This complication is:
    1. Neurological emergency
    2. Cardiac emergency
    3. Respiratory emergency
    4. Orthopedic emergency

    Answer: 3. Respiratory emergency

    Rationale: Once the diaphragm and intercostal muscles are affected by the progressive weakness of this disease, a respiratory emergency will ensue.

    Client need: Physiological integrity

    Nursing process: Evaluation

    Clinical skill level: 4

PARKINSON'S DISEASE

DEFINITION
A nervous disorder in which the patient exhibits extrapyramidal symptoms. The disease is chronic and progressively degenerative.

PATHOPHYSIOLOGY
A lack of dopamine in the basal ganglia.

ASSOCIATED MEDICAL CONDITIONS
- Bradykinesia
- Parkinsonian crisis

ASSESSMENT
- Muscle rigidity
- Tremor, pill-rolling of hands
- Fatigue
- Stone-faced expression
- Muscle cramps

CLIENT NEED
Physiological integrity

NURSING INTERVENTIONS
- Daily active and passive ROM exercises
- Monitor weight
- Administer antihistamines (Benadryl)
- Administer levodopa—converted from L dopa to dopamine in basal ganglia
- Administer laxatives and stool softeners
- Administer antidepressants if prescribed
- Administer eldepryl—inhibits dopamine breakdown
- Advise patient to maintain fluid intake of 2000 ml daily and moderate increase of dietary fiber

PATIENT TEACHING

- Stress importance of adhering to an exercise and walking program
- Instruct family to provide safe environment
- Teach patient and family the importance of taking medication exactly as prescribed
- Encourage active involvement in therapeutic program
- Encourage independence whenever possible

ASSOCIATED NURSING DIAGNOSES

- Anxiety
- Family coping, compromised, ineffective
- Hopelessness
- Pain, chronic
- Social isolation
- Fatigue
- Coping, ineffective individual
- Knowledge deficit
- Powerlessness

STUDY QUESTIONS

■ The medication prescribed for Parkinson's disease acts as a precursor to restore dopamine deficiency. What medication should the nurse give?
1. Dilantin
2. Ibuprofen
3. Tegretol
4. Levodopa

Answer: 4. Levodopa

Rationale: Levodopa is a synthetic precursor of dopamine and replaces the dopamine deficiency in Parkinson's. Dopamine cannot be given because it does not cross the blood-brain barrier.

Nursing process: Intervention

Client need: Physiological integrity

Clinical skill level: 2

■ Which is a response of the sympathetic nervous system to anxiety?
1. Tachycardia
2. Bradycardia
3. Constricted pupils
4. Increased peristalsis

Answer: 1. Tachycardia

Rationale: The sympathetic nervous system stimulates the body to response to stressors. The other body responses listed are actions of the sympathetic system.

Nursing process: Evaluation

Client need: Physiological integrity

Clinical skill level: 3

■ The nurse assesses a normal reflex when testing the plantar, or Babinski's, in an adult. What does she see?
1. Toes flaring upward
2. No obvious response
3. Toes bending downward
4. Sudden dorsal flexion

Answer: 3. Toes bending downward

Rationale: If the toes flare, and the foot turns upward, then the sign is positive and considered an abnormal finding in an adult.

Nursing process: Assessment

Client need: Physiological integrity

Clinical skill level: 2

■ During a neurological assessment, the nurse asks the patient to repeat a series of numbers. She is assessing:
1. Communication
2. Memory
3. Attention span
4. Thought process

Answer: 2. Memory

Rationale: Short-term memory can be easily assessed by asking the patient to repeat numbers or words.

Nursing process:

Client need: Physiological integrity

Clinical skill level: 2

■ The nurse asks a patient the time, his name, and date. She is assessing:
1. Cognitive ability
2. Intellectual ability
3. Level of consciousness
4. Past and present memory

Answer: 3. Level of consciousness

Rationale: The nurse is assessing orientation, a key component of the LOC assessment. If the patient responds positively to all three, then the nurse documents, oriented × 3.

Nursing process: Assessment

Client need: Physiological integrity

Clinical skill level: 1

UNIT 6
ENDOCRINE SYSTEM

- Diabetes Mellitus
- Hypothyroidism
- Syndrome of Inappropriate ADH Secretion (SIADH)

DIABETES MELLITUS

DEFINITION
Diabetes mellitus is a complex disease that alters protein, carbohydrates, and fat metabolism. It is classified into two stages: Type I or Type II. Type I is insulin dependent (IDDM) and Type II is non-insulin dependent (NIDDM).

PATHOPHYSIOLOGY
Type I is caused by a deficiency or lack of insulin that is normally produced by pancreatic beta cells. In Type II there is a deficiency of insulin as well as resistance by body tissues to bind to receptor sites on the surface of cells. Therefore, insulin is less effective in escorting glucose into the cells for use in the body.

ASSOCIATED MEDICAL CONDITIONS
- Hypertension
- Peripheral vascular disease

ASSESSMENT
- Polyuria
- Polyphagia
- Hypoglycemia
- Blurred vision
- Weight loss associated with increased food intake
- Polydipsia
- Dehydration
- Anxiety
- Nausea, vomiting
- Hyperglycemia (blood or urine)

CLIENT NEED
Physiological integrity

NURSING INTERVENTIONS
- Monitor blood glucose
- Teach to give self insulin injections
- Encourage regular exercise
- Provide emotional support
- Provide extensive nutritional education
- Administer insulin, if necessary

PATIENT TEACHING

- Teach patient how to monitor blood glucose
- Teach insulin rotation schedule
- Teach exercise regimen
- Teach patient American Diabetes Association (ADA) diet
- Teach to give self insulin injections
- Teach onset, peak and duration of insulin being prescribed
- Teach foot care

ASSOCIATED NURSING DIAGNOSES

- Activity intolerance, high risk for
- Denial, ineffective
- Anxiety
- Hopelessness
- Skin integrity, high risk for impaired
- Sexual patterns, altered
- Tissue perfusion, altered: peripheral
- Nutrition: more than body requirements, altered
- Home maintenance management, impaired
- Fatigue
- Infection, high risk for
- Noncompliance
- Sensory/perceptual alterations: visual, tactile
- Skin integrity, impaired
- Tissue integrity, impaired

STUDY QUESTIONS

■ A 16-year-old diabetic is planning to go to the movies with friends and wants to know what he can snack on at the movies. The nurse instructs the patient to:
1. Have a diet coke only
2. Sneak an apple in and count it as a fruit exchange
3. Explain to friends that he can't have anything to eat
4. Omit a bread and fat exchange during the day so he can have a small buttered popcorn

Answer: 4. Omit a bread and fat exchange during the day so he can have a small buttered popcorn.

Rationale: The purpose of the ADA food exchange list is to offer the diabetic patient a variety of foods.

Nursing process: Intervention

Client need: Physiological integrity

Clinical skill level: 3

■ While patient teaching with a diabetic, the nurse explains which pathophysiology causes diabetic retinopathy:
1. Adhesions
2. Hemorrhaging
3. Corneal abrasions
4. Optic edema

Answer: 2. Hemorrhaging

Rationale: Diabetic retinopathy is caused by the formation of micro-aneurysms in the retinal vessels, which leads to hemorrhaging.

Nursing process: Intervention

Client need: Physiological integrity

Clinical skill level: 2

■ The patient is in diabetic ketoacidosis. For which major complication must the nurse be alert?
1. Shock
2. Hypertension
3. High fever
4. Hypoglycemia

Answer: 1. Shock

Rationale: DKA causes dramatic depletion of intravascular volume, which causes hypotension and rapid heart rate. Other symptoms are weakness, headache, nausea, and abdominal pain.

Nursing process: Assessment

Client need: Physiological integrity

Clinical skill level: 3

■ When is a patient with Diabetes Mellitus, Type I, most vulnerable to ketoacidosis?
1. When fasting 2-3 days a week
2. When taking too much insulin
3. When under a lot of stress
4. When eating too many carbohydrates

Answer: 3. When under a lot of stress

Rationale: The body's demand for insulin is much greater during times of stress or illness. Since there is a lack of insulin in ketoacidosis, the deficiency is more dangerous.

Nursing process: Evaluation

Client need: Physiological integrity

Clinical skill level: 3

- In teaching a diabetic patient it is important initially to evaluate his:
    1. Dietary modification
    2. Understanding of the exchange list
    3. Ability to administer insulin
    4. Present understanding of diabetes

    Answer: 4. Present understanding of diabetes

    Rationale: The key to compliance is the patient's understanding of the disease and how he will cope with it. Self-regulation in diabetes is essential.

    Nursing process: Evaluation

    Client need: Physiological integrity

    Clinical skill level: 3

- The nurse teaches the diabetic patient that regular insulin peaks:
    1. 30 minutes
    2. 1 hour
    3. 2-4 hours
    4. 4-6 hours

    Answer: 3. 2-4 hours

    Rationale: Regular insulin is the short-acting insulin. Onset is ½-1 hour, peaks at 2-4 hours, and duration is 6-8 hours.

    Nursing process: Evaluation

    Client need: Physiological integrity

    Clinical skill level: 2

■ A diabetic patient develops pallor, cool skin, diaphoresis, and unconsciousness. In this emergency, the nurse prepares to administer:
1. D5W
2. Regular Insulin
3. Epinephrine
4. D_{50}

Answer: 4. D_{50}

Rationale: These are the signs and symptoms of severe hypoglycemia. The IV administration of 50% dextrose in water will have almost immediate effects. Caution: D_{50} is very irritating to the veins.

Nursing process: Intervention

Client need: Physiological integrity

Clinical skill level: 3

■ A diabetic patient is having abdominal surgery. Because of the medical history, the most common problem the nurse would expect is:
1. Risk of hemorrhaging
2. Fluid and electrolyte imbalances
3. Complications of anesthesia
4. Delayed wound healing

Answer: 4. Delayed wound healing

Rationale: Blood circulation is decreased in the diabetic patient, primarily caused by atherosclerotic plaques that appear to be more prominent in the diabetic disease process.

Nursing process: Outcome criteria

Client need: Physiological integrity

Clinical skill level: 3

- Before administration, insulin should:
    1. Always be refrigerated
    2. Be heated slowly
    3. Be divided into small doses
    4. Be warmed to room temperature

    Answer: 1. Always be refrigerated

    Rationale: If not refrigerated, insulin patency slowly decreases.

    Nursing process: Intervention

    Client need: Physiological integrity

    Clinical skill level: 1

- In planning patient teaching for a newly-diagnosed diabetic patient, the nurse knows that Type 1 diabetics are:
    1. Insulin dependent
    2. Not insulin dependent
    3. Suffering from complications of diabetes
    4. Usually diagnosed after age 40

    Answer: 1. Insulin dependent

    Rationale: Diabetes Mellitus is classified as Type I and Type II. Type I patients require insulin injections and Type II may be controlled with diet, exercise or oral hypoglycemias.

    Nursing process: Assessment

    Client need: Health promotion and maintenance

    Clinical skill level: 1

- If a diabetic is found unconscious and the nurse does not know the reason, the best intervention is:
  1. Treat for ketoacidosis
  2. Treat for insulin reaction
  3. Wait until blood glucose test results are evaluated
  4. Delay treating the patient until a physician arrives

  Answer: 2. Treat for insulin reaction

  Rationale: If the patient is unconscious, the problem most likely is insulin shock—emergency measures should be taken.

  Nursing process: Intervention

  Client need: Physiological integrity

  Clinical skill level: 3

- The patient with Diabetes Mellitus Type 1, should contact the physician immediately when a crisis occurs because he will:
  1. Gain weight rapidly
  2. Most likely experience insulin intolerance
  3. Need less insulin when he is ill
  4. Require more insulin in times of stress

  Answer: 4. Require more insulin in times of stress

  Rationale: During stressful periods, glucose levels rise because hormones such as epinephrine and cortisol tend to rise. Type I diabetics are at an increased risk for ketoacidosis.

  Nursing process: Evaluation

  Client need: Physiological integrity

  Clinical skill level: 3

- The patient is prescribed an intermediate-acting insulin. It is:
  1. PZI
  2. NPH
  3. Ultralente
  4. Semilente

  Answer: 2. NPH

  Rationale: NPH is the most common intermediate-acting insulin prescribed. The onset is 3-4 hours, the peak is 6-12 hours and the duration is 18-28 hours.

  Nursing process: Outcome criteria

  Client need: Physiological integrity

  Clinical skill level: 2

- A patient newly diagnosed with diabetes insipidus wants to know if he will have to take insulin. The nurse responds,"No. Diabetes insipidus is not caused by a lack of insulin, but by a lack of:
  1. ACTH."
  2. ADH."
  3. Glucose."
  4. Glucocorticoid."

  Answer: 2. ADH."

  Rationale: The deficiency of the anti-diuretic hormone causes excessive production of dilute urine.

  Nursing process: Intervention

  Client need: Physiological intervention

  Clinical skill level: 2

- When assessing a patient taking a sulfonylurea oral hypoglycemic agent, the nurse is aware that the medication that has the longest duration of action is:
  1. Regular insulin po
  2. Tolbutamide (orinase)
  3. Tolazamide (diabinese)
  4. Chlorpropamide (diabinese)

  Answer: 4. Chlorpropamide (diabinese)
  Rationale: Diabinese is one of the most common oral hypoglycemic prescribed to diabetic patients.
  Nursing process: Outcome criteria
  Client need: Health promotion and maintenance

  Clinical skill level: 3

HYPOTHYROIDISM

DEFINITION
Hypothyroidism occurs when there is a lack of thyroid hormone in the body's tissue. Severe hypothyroidism is called myxedema.

PATHOPHYSIOLOGY
A genetic link is suspected in this condition because there is evidence that it is transmitted by the X chromosome. (More women have it than men.) A deficiency of iodized salt is also considered a cause.

ASSOCIATED MEDICAL CONDITIONS
- Myxedema

ASSESSMENT
- Weakness
- Feelings of apathy, lethargy
- Puffy face and eyelids
- Loss of memory
- Impaired hearing
- Coarse hair
- Palpitations
- Anemia
- Slow speech (related to thickening of tongue)
- Flat affect
- Decreased cold tolerance
- Dry skin
- Poor wound healing
- Anxiety

NURSING INTERVENTIONS
- Administer thyroid hormone replacement (Levo-Thyroxine)
- Supportive psychological care, especially in regards to difficulty in communication

PATIENT TEACHING
- Functions of thyroid gland
- What happens physically when there is too much or too little thyroid hormone

- Do not take a "double dose" if a tablet is forgotten
- The generic and brand name of the medication
- Return for check-up as scheduled with the physician
- How and when to take medication, exactly as ordered
- Report any unusual symptoms

ASSOCIATED NURSING DIAGNOSES
- Body image disturbance
- Anxiety
- Hyperthermia
- Nutrition: potential for more than body requirements, altered
- Powerlessness
- Activity intolerance, high risk for
- Fatigue
- Knowledge deficit
- Physical mobility, impaired

STUDY QUESTIONS

■ The nurse is monitoring the patient who has been taking Levo-Thyroxine, 50 mg/daily for two weeks. What is one of the first indications that this drug is having the desired effect?

1. Reduced edema, weight loss
2. Weight gain, normal B/P
3. Brighter affect, weight gain
4. Weight loss, insomnia

Answer: 1. Reduced edema, weight loss

Rationale: This medication is very effective for the patient suffering hypothyroidism. It tends to be quite effective and initial results are the diuretic effects of the drug.

Client need: Physiological integrity

Nursing process: Planning

Clinical skill level: 4

■ When a child is born with a thyroid deficiency, the condition is:
1. Cushing's
2. Acromegaly
3. Dwarfism
4. Cretinism

Answer: 4. Cretinism

Rationale: Cretinism is the term used to describe a thyroid deficiency present at birth. In many cases, the mother may also suffer from the deficiency.

Nursing process: Assessment

Client need: Physiological integrity

Clinical skill level: 1

■ A post-thyroidectomy patient develops tetany. The nurse prepares to administer:
1. Valium IV
2. Protamine sulfate
3. Calcium gluconate
4. Magnesium sulfate

Answer: 3. Calcium gluconate

Rationale: Tetany can occur as a result of thyroid surgery when the parathyroid glands are accidentally removed or destroyed. Tetany is a shortage of calcium in the blood that causes muscle and nerves to twitch. Calcium gluconate is absorbed immediately and restores the blood to normal calcium levels.

Nursing process: Intervention

Client need: Physiological integrity

Clinical skill level: 3

■ A female patient, 34, has undergone a thyroidectomy. Two days post-op the nurse taps the patient on the cheek and watches for a muscle spasm in the cheek. This is the:
1. Kernig's sign
2. Chvostek's sign
3. Homan's sign
4. Trousseau's sign

Answer: 2. Chvostek's sign

Rationale: Chvostek's sign is a test to assess for hypocalcemia. If the spasm occurs, the calcium serum level is low. Hypocalcemia is a common complication post-thyroidectomy.

Nursing process: Assessment

Client need: Physiological integrity

Clinical skill level: 3

■ A female patient, 28, is diagnosed with hypothyroidism. She complains of:
1. Dry skin and chronic fatigue
2. Weight loss and insomnia
3. Uncontrollable emotions
4. Incontinence and fatigue

Answer: 1. Dry skin and chronic fatigue

Rationale: These are the most common symptoms, along with cold intolerance, of hypothyroidism.

Nursing process: Assessment

Rationale: Physiological integrity

Clinical skill level: 2

SIADH

Syndrome of Inappropriate ADH Secretion

DEFINITION
The excess secretion of the antidiuretic hormone from the pituitary gland. The consequence is inappropriate reabsorption of water in the renal tubules. In the patient, therefore, the water is retained.

PATHOPHYSIOLOGY
SIADH is not always an endocrine disorder but can occur in several disorders such as cancer, pneumonia, head injury and the intake of some medications. When the body is altered due to pulmonary disease, malignant tumors, infections or dysfunctions of the central nervous system, the body may respond with increased ADH production which leads to SIADH. Example: When cardiac output is decreased, ADH secretion increases so that blood volume will also increase.

MOST COMMON MEDICAL CONDITIONS
- Trauma
- Infection
- Pneumothorax
- Meningitis
- Pneumonia
- Cerebral hemorrhage
- Head injury

ASSESSMENT
- Edema
- Decreased urinary output
- Muscle cramping
- Weight gain even though anorexic
- Confusion
- Nausea and vomiting
- Monitor for hyponatremia

CLIENT NEED
Physiological integrity

NURSING INTERVENTIONS
- Strict I&O
- Weight (daily)
- Restrict fluids, according to orders
- Administer oral Lasix (furosemide) (to ensure excretion of dilute urine)
- Vital signs
- Monitor urine chemistry
- Administer demeclocycline (an antibiotic)

PATIENT TEACHING
- Need for fluid restriction
- Ability to recognize electrolyte imbalances and need to notify health care provider of such imbalances.
- Foods that are high in potassium
  - Bananas
- Take medication at times prescribed, especially Lasix
- Importance of maintaining special diet: Low or high sodium depending on whether acute or chronic hyponatremia is present.

ASSOCIATED NURSING DIAGNOSES
- Cardiac output, decreased
- Nutrition: less than body requirements, altered
- Fluid volume excess
- Urinary elimination, altered

STUDY QUESTIONS

■ A nursing intervention in caring for the patient with SIADH is:
1. Force fluids
2. Restrict salt
3. Restrict food intake
4. Restrict fluids

Answer: 4. Restrict fluids

Rationale: General management of SIADH involves restricting fluids because retained water is very slowly excreted.

Nursing process: Intervention

Client need: Physiological integrity

> Clinical skill level: 4

■ The electrolyte imbalance the nurse must assess in the patient with SIADH is:
1. Hypernatremia
2. Hyponatremia
3. Hypokalemia
4. Hyperkalemia

Answer: 2. Hyponatremia

Rationale: Because the patient experiences difficulty excreting urine that has been diluted during the reabsorption process, hyponatremia develops. Symptoms include nausea, muscle cramping, abdominal discomfort, and weakness.

Nursing process: Assessment

Client need: Physiological integrity

> Clinical skill level: 4

GENERAL STUDY QUESTIONS

■ Cortisol replacement may be ordered for the patient following a transsphenoidal hypophysectomy. The nurse monitors for hypotension, fever, nausea, and vomiting. These are signs and symptoms of:
1. Thyroid storm
2. Addisonian crisis
3. ACTH crisis
4. Cushing's crisis

Answer: 2. Addisonian crisis

Rationale: This condition, also known as adrenal crisis, produces hyponatremia and hyperkalemia. If allowed to progress, it could be fatal.

Nursing process: Assessment

Client need: Physiological integrity

Clinical skill level: 3

■ Another important component in the care of a patient with diabetes insipidus is:
1. Daily weight
2. Early ambulation
3. Nutrition education
4. Glucose monitoring

Answer: 1. Daily weight

Rationale: A weight gain of 1 lb indicates fluid retention of approximately 50 ml. If there is a weight gain of more that 1-2 lbs/day, this could indicate excessive fluid intake and retention and should be reported immediately to the physician.

Nursing process: Intervention

Client need: Physiological integrity

Clinical skill level: 3

■ In planning the care of a patient with diabetes insipidus, a priority must be prevention of:
1. Foot ulcers
2. Excessive fluid intake
3. High blood glucose
4. Excessive food intake

Answer: 2. Excessive fluid intake

Rationale: One of the symptoms this patient experiences is extreme thirst and excessive fluid intake can easily become a habit that the nurse must attempt to control.

Nursing process: Intervention

Client need: Physiological integrity

Clinical skill level: 3

■ The nurse does a mental status assessment on the patient undergoing the Dexamethasone Suppression Test to diagnose Cushing's Syndrome. Which psychological problem might alter this test?
1. Schizophrenia
2. Bulimia
3. Depression
4. Drug abuse

Answer: 3. Depression

Rationale: Severe depression may produce a false positive because a patient suffering depression may show an elevated morning cortisol level.

Nursing process: Evaluation

Client need: Physiological integrity

Clinical skill level: 4

- The nurse is doing an initial history and assessment on the patient newly diagnosed with aldosteronism. The nurse asks the patient about ingestion of:
    1. Milk products
    2. Eggs
    3. Licorice
    4. Pizza

    Answer: 3. Licorice

    Rationale: Licorice has mild mineralocorticoid properties and, when ingested in large amounts, can cause excess of mineralocorticoids.

    Nursing Process: Assessment

    Client Need: Physiological integrity

    Clinical skill level: 4

- Hypertension is a common sign in the diagnosis of aldosteronism. What is the other major clinical finding that is paired with hypertension when this disorder is diagnosed?
    1. Hyperkalemia
    2. Hypokalemia
    3. Hypernatremia
    4. Hyponatremia

    Answer: 2. Hypokalemia

    Rationale: There is no apparent cause for the hypokalemia, such as diuretics or diarrhea.

    Nursing Process: Assessment

    Client Need: Physiological integrity

    Clinical skill level: 4

- The nursing assessment states a patient has a "cushingoid" appearance. Which of these signs does this term describe?
    1. Buffalo hump, moon face
    2. Evenly distributed body fat
    3. Obesity, hirsutism
    4. Osteoporosis, truncal obesity

    Answer: 1. Buffalo hump, moon face

    Rationale: The increased fat deposits that cause "buffalo humps" and moon faces are cardinal signs of Cushing's disease. The reason for the unusual distribution of fat is not known.

    Nursing Process: Assessment

    Client Need: Physiological integrity

    Clinical skill level: 3

- Perioperative management for the patient having surgery to remove an aldosterone secreting adenoma is focused on:
    1. Blood pressure
    2. Urine output
    3. Pulse pressure
    4. Respiratory rate

    Answer: 1. Blood pressure

    Rationale: The blood pressure may be unstable—and hypertension is a common complication—related to changes in aldosterone levels. In addition, if the patient begins to experience an adrenal crisis, hypotension would be one of the first signs of this complication.

    Nursing process: Assessment

    Client need: Physiological integrity

    Clinical skill level

■ A 32-year-old woman is diagnosed with Addison's disease. She states, "I've never heard of that before. What causes it?" The nurse replies:
1. "No one knows. It's a real mystery."
2. "A decrease in hormones called the adrenocortical hormones."
3. "High blood pressure and obesity."
4. "Too much aldosterone and the antidiuretic hormone."

Answer: 2. "A decrease in hormones called the adrenocortical hormones."

Rationale: Decreased levels of glucocorticords and mineralocorticords, both adrenocortical hormones, cause Addison's disease.

Nursing process: Intervention

Client need: Physiological integrity

Clinical skill level: 2

■ Hyperthyroid patients generally exhibit which one of the following symptoms?
1. Weight loss
2. Constipation
3. Thickened skin
4. Lower body temperature

Answer: 1. Weight loss

Rationale: Anorexia is often a symptom of hyperthyroidism and should be treated with a diet high in calories and vitamins.

Nursing process: Assessment

Client need: Physiological integrity

Clinical skill level:3

■ When caring for the patient who has had surgery for a pituitary adenoma, what special instructions should be emphasized?
1. Be careful taking a shower
2. Keep the dressing dry
3. Do not brush your teeth
4. Do not sit up in bed

Answer: 3. Do not brush your teeth

Rationale: Brushing teeth is contraindicated because the suture line is made between the upper gums and lips.

Nursing process: Interventions

Client need: Physiological integrity

Clinical skill level: 2

■ A female, 28, is admitted with vague complaints of nervousness and restlessness. She states she occasionally experiences jerky movements and cries without reason. The nurse suspects a thyroid disorder and closely assesses the:
1. Reflexes
2. Teeth and gums
3. Tongue
4. Eyes

Answer: 4. Eyes.

Rationale: The nurse should assess this patient for exophthalmos, a condition common in Grave's disease. It is the protrusion of the eyeballs that produces a blank stare.

Nursing process: Assessment

Client need: Physiological integrity

Clinical skill level: 2

- The nurse assesses severe exophthalmos in a patient diagnosed with Grave's disease. What major complications threaten if not treated aggressively?
  1. Infection
  2. Cataracts and decreasing sight
  3. Ulceration and blindness
  4. Brain damage and blindness

  Answer: 3. Ulceration and decreasing sight

  Rationale: In severe hyperthyroidism, edema prevents the eye closing, resulting in lid retraction. The eye becomes dry and susceptible to injury.

  Nursing process: Evaluation

  Client Need: Physiological integrity

  Clinical skill level: 3

- The patient with hypercalcemia should be closely monitored with ECG as well as the serum calcium levels. The nurse should watch for:
  1. Missing T wave
  2. Shortened QT interval
  3. Lengthened QT interval
  4. Tachycardia and palpations

  Answer: 2. Shortened QT interval

  Rationale: Life-threatening cardiac dysrhythmias may occur in severe hypercalcemia.

  Nursing process: Assessment

  Client need: Physiological integrity

  Clinical skill level: 4

■ The patient diagnosed with primary hyperparathyroidism is encouraged to drink at least 3L/day. The rationale for forcing fluids is to prevent the complication of:
1. Hypertension and MI
2. Hemorrhage and hypotension
3. Infection and renal stones
4. Dropping B/P and pulse

Answer: 3. Infection and renal stones

Rationale: A patient with this diagnosis is experiencing hypercalcemia, often severe. Hypercalcemia causes the urine to be alkaline, increasing the risk of urinary tract infections. the increased calcium levels put this patient at a higher risk of renal stones. The threat of both complications is reduced if urine is dilute.

Nursing Process: Evaluation

Client Need: Physiological integrity

Clinical skill level: 4

■ The nurse assesses the patient with primary hyperparathyroidism has high levels of serum calcium and a shortened QT interval. She calls the physician and prepares to administer:
1. Lidocaine
2. Procardine
3. Lactated Ringer's
4. Normal saline IV

Answer: 4. Normal saline IV

Rationale: Normal saline will increase the circulating volume in an attempt to decrease calcium levels. Normal saline infusion will cause a saline diuresis. When sodium is excreted, calcium is excreted.

Nursing process: Intervention

Client need: Physiological integrity

Clinical skill level: 4

- In planning the care of the patient with hyperparathyroidism, safety is a priority concern. These patients are at an increased risk for fractures because they suffer:
    1. High calcium levels
    2. Weakness and fatigue
    3. Loss of eye sight
    4. Cardiac dysrhythmias

    Answer: 2. Weakness and fatigue

    Rationale: Weakness and fatigue are cardinal symptoms of hypercalcemia.

    Nursing process: Evaluation

    Client need: Physiological integrity

    Clinical skill level: 4

- The antidiuretic hormone (ADH) is secreted by the:
    1. Kidneys
    2. Adrenals
    3. Anterior pituitary
    4. Posterior pituitary

    Answer: 4. Posterior pituitary

    Rationale: The ADH is synthesized in the hypothalamus and moves down the nerve cells linking to the posterior pituitary gland, which stores them. When blood pressure decreases or osmality of the blood increases, ADH is secreted.

    Nursing process: Assessment

    Client need: Health promotion and maintenance

    Clinical skill level: 2

■ An eosinophilic tumor of the pituitary gland causes gigantism in a child, and in the adult it results in:
   1. Acromegaly
   2. Hypopituitarism
   3. Cushing's syndrome
   4. Atrophy of the sex organs

Answer: 1. Acromegaly

Rationale: Acromegaly is the enlargement of the jaw, face, feet and hands in adults due to the overproduction of hormones of the pituitary gland. In children, this disorder is rare since overproduction of the growth hormone in children results in the enlargement of the long bones which have not stopped growing yet because of their young age.

Nursing process: Assessment

Client need: Physiological integrity

Clinical skill level: 3

UNIT 7
MUSCULOSKELETAL SYSTEM

- Cast
- Compartment Syndrome
- Fractures
- Osteoarthritis
- Osteomyelitis
- Traction

CAST

DEFINITION
An immobilizing device that is molded to the specific body part that is being treated.

TYPES OF CASTS
- There are two types of casts, plaster and fiberglass.
- Characteristics of a plaster cast:
  - When wet (newly-applied) gives off heat; cools in about 15 minutes
  - Full strength when dry
  - Must be handled carefully with the palm of the hand (fingertip may cause indentations which, in turn, may cause ulcerations)
  - Requires 24-72 hours to dry
  - Cannot be exposed to water or hydrotherapy
- Characteristics of fiberglass cast:
  - Lighter weight than plaster
  - Very durable and water resistant
  - Becomes rigid in a few minutes
  - Can be exposed to water and hydrotherapy
  - Fewer ulcerations than with plastic, but allergic reactions to fiberglass may cause rash.

ASSOCIATED MEDICAL CONDITIONS
- Fractures
- Sprains

ASSESSMENT
- Neurovascular checks
- Peripheral pulses
- Degree of bruising
- Dry cast should be white, shiny, firm, odorless, resonant
- Edema
- Pain
- Lacerations or abrasions

CLIENT NEED
Physiological integrity

NURSING INTERVENTIONS
- Provide support to distal part of extremity to be casted
- Support cast with palm of hands while drying
- Administer pain medication
- Keep extremity elevated above heart level
- Encourage isometric exercises every hour
- Expose newly-applied cast to air; do not cover

PATIENT TEACHING
- Do not scratch under cast (may cause ulcerations)
- Keep extremity elevated
- Do not put anything in cast
- For plaster cast:
  - Keep cast dry
- For fiberglass cast:
  - If cast gets wet, dry thoroughly with hair dryer on cool setting
- If cast tightens around skin, notify physician immediately
- Teach isometric exercises
- Report any odor to physician immediately

ASSOCIATED NURSING DIAGNOSES
- Activity intolerance
- Disuse syndrome, high risk for
- Injury, high risk for
- Peripheral neurovascular dysfunction, high risk for
- Skin integrity, high risk for impaired
- Constipation
- Home maintenance management, impaired
- Pain
- Physical mobility, impaired
- Tissue perfusion, altered (peripheral)

STUDY QUESTIONS

■ The nurse notes according to the chart, the patient who has a cast had been complaining of pain over a bony prominence. However, during the last 8 hours the patient has not complained of pain. The nurse suspects:
1. The patient was imagining the pain
2. The pain was only temporary
3. The swelling is decreasing
4. An ulceration has probably occurred

Answer: 4. An ulceration has probably occurred

Rationale: Pain is the warning of a threatening pressure ulcer, but once the ulceration breaks the skin the pain decreases or disappears.

Nursing process: Evaluation

Client need: Physiological integrity

Clinical skill level: 3

■ The patient with a leg cast complains of persistent itching. The best nursing intervention is:
1. Notify the physician immediately
2. Apply topical medication under cast
3. Apply cool air from hair dryer
4. Tell patient to ask doctor for medication

Answer: 3. Apply cool air from hair dryer

Rationale: Itching under the cast is a common complaint, and cool air will somewhat alleviate this symptom.

Nursing process: Intervention

Client need: Physiological integrity

Clinical skill level: 2

■ The patient with a leg cast complains of numbness, tingling and burning pain. The nurse assesses pressure around the fibula. The complication the nurse should assess is:
1. Footdrop
2. Compartment syndrome
3. Bone infection
4. Volkmann's contracture

Answer: 1. Footdrop

Rationale: Pressure on the fibula results in injury to the peroneal nerve, which, in turn, causes footdrop. The complication is often irreversible.

Nursing process: Assessment

Client need: Physiological integrity

> Clinical skill level: 3

■ The nurse assesses increasing anxiety, increased respiratory and pulse rate, and elevated blood pressure in a patient with a spica cast. The nurse evaluates that this patient is experiencing cast syndrome. The danger of this complication is:
1. Ileus
2. Constipation
3. Vomiting
4. Panic attacks

Answer: 1. Ileus

Rationale: With immobility, a decrease in gastrointestinal motility occurs. The patient experiences distention, nausea and vomiting. A window may be cut over the abdominal area to release the pressure on the superior mesenteric artery.

Nursing process: Intervention

Client need: Physiological integrity

> Clinical skill level: 3

COMPARTMENT SYNDROME

DEFINITION
Swelling occurs around a constrictive device or dressing, causing tissue anoxia. This results in severe pain, loss of mobility, and sensory function.

PATHOPHYSIOLOGY
Increasing presssure on tissue, usually within a small space, impairs circulation which causes damage to the entrapped nerves.

ASSOCIATED MEDICAL CONDITIONS
- Fractures that require casts
- Dislocations
- Sprains that require splints

ASSESSMENT
- Neuromuscular assessment:
  - Numbness, especially in extremity
  - Tingling, especially in extremity
  - Pain (burning indicates pressure, muscle spasm)
  - Skin color, especially pallor, cyanosis, dusky tone
  - Pulse, especially distal to injury
  - Capillary refill (return to normal in 3 seconds)
  - Edema
  - Is immobilizing device (such as cast or splint) constricting? There should be at least one cm space between skin and device
- Unrelieved pain
- Increased swelling around resistive device
- Poor capillary refill
- Paralysis in affected extremity

CLIENT NEED
Physiological integrity

NURSING INTERVENTIONS
- Neurovascular checks every hour
- Perform passive ROM, if indicated
- Encourage mobility, active ROM
- Encourage isometric exercises (to maintain muscle strength)

PATIENT TEACHING
- Specifically, what function can be provided and what is prohibited
- How to take pain medications and side-effects that may occur
- Signs and symptoms of pain and edema should be reported to the physician
- ROM exercises are essential even though extremity appears immobile

ASSOCIATED NURSING DIAGNOSES
- Activity intolerance
- Disuse syndrome, high risk for
- Injury, high risk for
- Tissue perfusion, altered (peripheral)
- Pain
- Constipation
- Home maintenance management, impaired
- Physical mobility, impaired
- Management of therapeutic regime (individual), ineffective
- Self-care deficit: bathing/hygiene, dressing/grooming, feeding, toileting

STUDY QUESTIONS

■ The patient who has an arm cast is complaining of pain that cannot be relieved. He also states that he is not able to move the fingers on the affected extremity. The nurse assesses increased swelling around the cast. These signs and symptoms are evaluated as:
1. Part of the injury
2. Normal reaction to a cast
3. Allergic reaction to cast
4. Compartment syndrome

Answer: 4. Compartment syndrome

Rationale: Unrelieved pain and paralysis are cardinal symptoms of compartment syndrome.

Nursing process: Evaluation

Client need: Physiological integrity

|Clinical skill level: 2|

■ The patient who has a cast on the right arm has just been diagnosed with compartment syndrome. The nurse prepares:
1. For surgery stat
2. To bivalve cast
3. To wrap with ACE
4. To administer Valium IV

Answer: 2. To bivalve cast

Rationale: The cast must be cut in two to relieve the pressure, and the extremity must be elevated. If these two actions do not relieve the pressure and edema, then a fasciotomy may be considered.

Nursing process: Intervention

Client need: Physiological integrity

|Clinical skill level: 3|

FRACTURES

DEFINITION
A fracture is a break in the bone.

PATHOPHYSIOLOGY
Fractures usually occur from a force or blow to the bone that the bone cannot absorb. Breaks in the bone also occur spontaneously in bone that is weakened by osteoporosis and cancer.

Types of Fractures
- Complete:
  - The bone is broken through.
- Incomplete
  - Bone is broken through only part of the bone. Example is the greenstick fracture that usually occurs in children.
- Simple
  - The broken bone is not projecting through the skin.
- Open
  - The broken bone breaks the skin and protrudes. Also called a compound fracture.
- Displaced
  - The broken bone is out of its normal position.
- Comminuted
  - The bone is broken into three or more fragments.
- Compression
  - A bone, such as a vertebrae, collapses.
- Depressed
  - The bone, such as in a skull fracture, is pushed in.
- Impacted
  - The ends of the broken bone are jammed into each other.

ASSOCIATED MEDICAL CONDITIONS
- Fractured hips
- Cervical fracture
- Compound fracture
- Osteoporosis
- Fractured ribs
- Pelvic fracture
- Cancer

ASSESSMENT
- Pain at site of injury
- Muscle spasms
- Limited physical mobility
- Alignment, obvious deformity
- Ecchymosis
- Edema
- Laceration of the soft tissue
- Lack of stability in movement
- Bleeding, as in a compound fracture

CLIENT NEED
Physiological integrity

NURSING INTERVENTIONS
- Immobilize affected part
- Prepare for x-rays
- Administer Valium IV for muscle spasms
- Administer pain medications
- Stop bleeding

PATIENT TEACHING
- Activity intolerance
- Fatigue
- Infection, high risk for
- Pain
- Post trauma response
- Skin integrity, high risk for
- Anxiety
- Body image disturbance
- Injury, high risk for
- Physical mobility, impaired
- Role performance, altered
- Tissue perfusion, altered: peripheral

ASSOCIATED NURSING DIAGNOSES
- Activity intolerance
- Home maintenance management, impaired
- Self care deficit: Bathing/Hygiene, Dressing/Grooming, Feeding/Toileting
- Infection, high risk for
- Peripheral neurovascular dysfunction, high risk for
- Pain, chronic

STUDY QUESTIONS

■ The elderly patient has just sustained a fractured hip, and Buck's traction is in place. The nurse suspects the femoral artery may have been torn in the fall. The patient must be closely monitored for signs and symptoms of:
1. Cardiac arrest
2. Cerebrovascular accident
3. Hypovolemic shock
4. Narcotic overdose from medications

Answer: 3. Hypovolemic shock

Rationale: The internal blood loss from a hip fracture may quickly reach hemorrhagic proportions, and if a major vessel such as the femoral artery is also damaged the patient is at a high risk for hypovolemic shock.

Nursing process: Assessment

Client need: Physiological integrity

Clinical skill level: 4

■ The first priority of care for the patient who has just sustained a fractured hip is:
1. Start IV
2. Administer narcotic IM
3. Give po pain medication
4. Immobilize extremity

Answer: 4. Immobilize extremity

Rationale: The first priority should be to immobilize the affected extremity, with Buck's traction, to avoid any further damage to the surrounding tissue and to control pain and decrease muscle spasms.

Nursing process: Intervention

Client need: Physiological integrity

Clinical skill level: 2

■ The greatest danger to the patient with long-bone fractures in ICU is:
1. Fat embolism
2. Internal bleeding
3. Pulmonary edema
4. Cardiac arrest

Answer: 1. Fat embolism
Rationale: Fat embolism is a complication that develops 48-72 hours post-fracture, especially of the long bones. It is a respiratory emergency.
Nursing process: Assessment
Client need: Physiological integrity

Clinical skill level: 3

■ What is the priority nursing action required when the nurse assesses an impending fat embolism?
1. Administer Valium IV push to calm restlessness
2. For hypovolemic emergency, administer 1000 cc D_5W
3. For respiratory emergency, administer oxygen
4. For cardiac emergency, administer pint of blood

Answer: 3. For respiratory emergency, administer oxygen
Rationale: Fat embolism is a respiratory emergency, and oxygen should be administered immediately.
Nursing process: Intervention
Client need: Physiological integrity

Clinical skill level: 2

■ The patient suffering a hip fracture has been prescribed Valium 10 mg IM every 4 hours. What is the rationale for administering this medication?
1. To relieve pain
2. To relieve anxiety
3. To relieve muscle spasms
4. To potentiate narcotics

Answer: 3. To relieve muscle spasms

Rationale: Valium was originally introduced as a muscle relaxant, then became popular as an anti-anxiety agent.

Nursing process: Intervention

Client need: Physiological integrity

Clinical skill level: 2

■ A young man suffers a compound fracture of the tibula-fibula in a motorcycle accident. There is also a question of head injury because he ws not wearing a helmet. The emergency room nurse prepares to give:
1. Demerol IM
2. Morphine IV
3. Mannitol IV
4. Tetanus toxid

Answer: 4. Tetanus toxid

Rationale: A tetanus toxid is required for contaminated open wounds that occur outside of the home. Narcotics would be contraindicated with head injuries. Mannitol would be ordered only with increasing intracranial pressure.

Nursing process: Intervention

Client need: Physiological integrity

Clinical skill level: 4

OSTEOARTHRITIS

DEFINITION
Osteoarthritis is a degenerative joint disease characterized by progressive loss of cartilage and changes on the bone at the joint margins. It is a non-inflammatory disorder.

PATHOPHYSIOLOGY
The most significant pathologies are destruction of cartilage and bony formations at the edge of the joints. Contributing factors are obesity, trauma, or other joint problems.

ASSOCIATED MEDICAL CONDITIONS
Degenerative joint disease

ASSESSMENT
- Gait
- Stiffness (early a.m. until about an hour after rising)
- Muscle spasms
- ROM
- Side effects to pain medication
- Bony nodules:
  - Herberden's nodes (distal interphalangeal joints)
  - Bouchard's nodes (proximal interphalangeal joints)
- Mobility
- Pain (worse with activity—most common symptom)
- Crepitus
- Joint swelling

CLIENT NEED
Physiological integrity

NURSING INTERVENTIONS
- Apply moist heat to relieve stiffness
- Active/passive ROM to relieve stiffness
- Administer pain medication

- Monitor skin for breakdown
- Treat symptoms of pain and stiffness
- Schedule daily routine for adequate rest and activity
- Monitor for side-effects of non-narcotic pain medication

PATIENT TEACHING

- Teach weight loss diet, if appropriate
- Exercises to encourage physical therapy
- Teach appropriate use of devices, such as walkers, canes and crutches
- Do not exercise joints if painful or swollen
- Occupational therapy
- Teach self-care related to pain management
- Daily routine including rest, heat or cold therapy and positioning

ASSOCIATED NURSING DIAGNOSES

- Activity intolerance, high risk for
- Fatigue
- Pain, chronic
- Role performance, altered
- Coping, ineffective individual
- Home maintenance management, impaired
- Physical mobility, impaired
- Self-care deficit: bathing/hygiene, dressing/grooming, feeding, toileting

STUDY QUESTIONS

■ When teaching a patient to use the walker, the nurse instructs the patient to:
1. Take a step then move the walker forward
2. Grip the walker with dominant hand only
3. Move the walker forward while taking a step
4. Move walker only after both feet have moved

Answer: 3. Move the walker forward while taking a step

Rationale: This is the safest technique to teach when the patient is using a walker to prevent loss of balance or tripping.

Nursing process: Intervention

Client need: Safe, effective care environment

Clinical skill level: 2

■ A patient is being taught how to use crutches. He is measured for crutches and placement of the handgrips has been determined. The nurse should verify that the distance between the crutch pad and the axilla is:
1. 1 to 2 inches
2. 3 to 4 inches
3. 1 to 2 finger widths
4. 1 ½ to 2 inches

Answer: 4. 1 ½ to 2 inches

Rationale: This is the optimal position for movement as well as prevention of irritation to the axilla.

Nursing process: Intervention

Client need: Physiological integrity

Clinical skill level: 2

■ The patient with osteoarthritis asks the nurse, "What kind of disease is this anyway?" The nurse explains this is:
1. An inflammatory process
2. An autoimmune disorder
3. A degenerative disease
4. An incurable, malignant disease

Answer: 3. A degenerative process

Rationale: Osteoarthritis occurs commonly after "wear and tear" on weight bearing joints, causing hypertrophic changes in the joints.

Nursing process: Assessment

Client need: Physiological integrity

Clinical skill level: 2

■ There are major differences between aspirin and acetaminophen (Tylenol). Among them are:
1. Tylenol has only a weak anti-inflammatory response
2. Tylenol overdose is not as dangerous as aspirin
3. Tylenol is much less expensive than aspirin
4. Tylenol is contraindicated in children

Answer: 1. Tylenol has only a weak anti-inflammatory response

Rationale: Aspirin has a strong anti-inflammatory action, whereas Tylenol is an analgesic with some anti-pyretic qualities but not the kind of anti-inflammatory action that aspirin has.

Nursing process: Outcome criteria

Client need: Physiological integrity

Clinical skill level: 2

OSTEOMYELITIS

DEFINITION
Osteomyelitis is a term describing any bone infection. While generally originating in bacteria, osteomyelitis may also be caused by viral or fungal infections. The organisms may be introduced directly into the bone or may be spread from soft tissue or travel through the blood.

PATHOPHYSIOLOGY
Staphylococcus aureaus is the most common infecting organism in osteomyelitis. Indirect entry osteomyelitis usually affects growing bone in boys—particularly the long leg bones—and is associated with local trauma. Direct entry osteomyelitis occurs when an open wound is present. The bacteria enters through the blood supply and lodges in an area where circulation is slow. As the bacteria grows, it creates pressure which leads to ischemia. The bone then dies, and the dead area separates from the living area to form sequestra where the bacteria continue to thrive.

ASSESSMENT
- Erythema
- Fever (often above 101°)
- Heat
- Localized pain or tenderness
- Swelling around affected bone
- History of recent trauma

CLIENT NEED
Physiological integrity

NURSING INTERVENTIONS
- Assist in sequestrectomy to remove dead bone
- Administer antibiotics 4 to 6 weeks as ordered
- Psychological support
- Needle aspiration/percutaneous needle biopsy to relieve pressure
- Frequent position changes to promote comfort

PATIENT TEACHING

- Wound care
- Diet high in protein, Vitamin C
- Need for rest
- Importance of taking medication as ordered

ASSOCIATED NURSING DIAGNOSES

- Activity intolerance, high risk for
- Anxiety
- Pain
- Disuse syndrome, high risk for
- Fatigue
- Self care deficit: bathing/hygiene, dressing/grooming, feeding/toileting

STUDY QUESTIONS

■ A young man, 26, was hospitalized following an auto accident 6 days ago. He now has a temperature of 102.4° F. The nurse prepares to administer, per doctor's orders:

1. Narcotic medication
2. Russell's traction
3. PO antibiotics
4. IV antibiotics

Answer: 4. IV antibiotics

Rationale: Osteomyelitis is an infection of the bone that is very difficult to heal and potent IV antibiotics are prescribed in the aggressive treatment of this disorder.

Nursing process: Intervention

Client need: Physiological integrity

Clinical skill level: 3

■ A 24-year-old man is admitted with a fever of 102.4° and pain and edema in the right hip. He states he has had a low grade fever for "about a week." He denies any history of trauma, but states he does play handball and constantly hits his right hip against the wall. This assessment is indicative of:
   1. Osteoarthritis
   2. Osteomyelitis
   3. Osteomalacia
   4. Osteoporosis

   Answer: 3. Osteomyelitis
   Rationale: The cardinal signs of bone infection are fever, pain and edema in the affected extremity.
   Nursing process: Assessment
   Client need: Physiological integrity

   Clinical skill level: 3

■ Adequate nutritional status is essential for the patient with osteomyelitis. Emphasis is on foods high in:
   1. Potassium and zinc
   2. Calcium and phosphorus
   3. Calcium and Vitamin D
   4. Protein, Vitamin C, calories

   Answer: 4. Protein, Vitamin C, calories
   Rationale: Protein and Vitamin C are required for healing, and calories are needed related to the energy that the fever will burn.
   Nursing process: Intervention
   Client need: Physiological integrity

   Clinical skill level : 3

TRACTION

DEFINITION
Traction is the pulling force applied to the body to control muscle spasms, to immobilize a fracture, to reduce a fracture, or to straighten a deformity.

TYPES OF TRACTION
- Straight
  - Buck's extension
  - Pelvic extension
- Skin
  - Buck's extension
  - Russell's traction
- Skeletal
  - Kirschner wire
  - Steinmann's Pin
  - Crutchfield tongs
  - Gardner-Wells tongs
- Balance
  - Thomas splint with Pearson attachment
- Manual
  - Temporary traction applied by using the hands

ASSOCIATED MEDICAL CONDITIONS
- Dislocation of the hip
- Fractures

ASSESSMENT
- Proper alignment
- Neurovascular status:
  - Capillary refill
  - Color
  - Temperature
  - Mobility
  - Edema
  - Pulses

- Skin integrity
- Sensory deprivation (confusion, disorientation)
- Homan's sign
- Pressure ulcers
- Breath sounds (for congestion and pneumonia)
- Constipation

CLIENT NEED
Physiological integrity

NURSING INTERVENTIONS
- Never interrupt skeletal traction
- Ensure that weights and ropes hand free, without obstruction
- Maintain line of pull
- Administer prescribed muscle relaxants
- Do not remove or alter weights from traction
- Maintain countertraction (body weight or bed position are examples of countertraction)
- Prescribe pain medications
- Encourage fluids and high fiber diet

PATIENT TEACHING
- Purpose of traction
- High fiber diet
- Importance of proper alignment

ASSOCIATED NURSING DIAGNOSES
- Activity intolerance
- Constipation
- Disuse syndrome, high risk for
- Hopelessness
- Noncompliance
- Skin integrity, high risk for impaired
- Tissue perfusion, altered (peripheral)
- Anxiety
- Fatigue
- Home maintenance, impaired
- Knowledge deficit
- Pain, chronic
- Peripheral neurovascular dysfunction, high risk for

STUDY QUESTIONS

■ In applying pelvic traction, the nurse teaches the patient that the belt goes around the:
1. Buttocks
2. Waist
3. Iliac crest
4. Lower diaphragm

Answer: 3. Iliac crest
Rationale: The purpose of pelvic traction is to pull the pelvis and lower spine into proper alignment.
Nursing process: Intervention
Client need: Physiological integrity

Clinical skill level: 2

■ When cleansing pin sites, the crust that forms around the site should be left intact until the skin is healed and it sloughs off. The one exception to this is if there is underlying evidence of:
1. Granulation
2. Bleeding
3. Infection
4. Muscle tear

Answer: 3. Infection
Rationale: If edema, erythema, odor or drainage is noted at the pin site, the curst should be removed with hydrogen peroxide, and the wound cleansed as thoroughly as possible.
Nursing process: Intervention
Client need: Physiological integrity

Clinical skill level: 3

- How often should the nurse document neurocirculatory status in a patient in traction?
    1. Every 15 minutes
    2. Every 20 minutes
    3. Every two hours
    4. Every four hours

    Answer: 3. Every two hours

    Rationale: Neurocirculatory complications can begin quickly without warning. Signs of problems include edema, pain and inability to move extremity.

    Nursing process: Intervention

    Client need: Physiological integrity

    Clinical skill level: 3

- The patient in Buck's traction complains of pain on the top of the affected leg and inability to move toes. The nurse assesses a slight drop of the foot. She evaluates this as:
    1. Normal discomfort when in traction
    2. Normal positioning for Buck's
    3. Contracture of the affected leg
    4. Peroneal nerve compression

    Answer: 4. Peroneal nerve compression

    Rationale: Pressure over the peroneal nerve is common. With early assessment, the extremity can be elevated, the foot positioned properly and the footdrop prevented.

    Client need: Physiological integrity

    Nursing process: Intervention

    Clinical skill level: 4

UNIT 8
URINARY/RENAL SYSTEM

- Pyelonephritis
- Renal Calculi
- Urinary Tract Infections
- Renal Failure

PYELONEPHRITIS

DEFINITION
Pyelonephritis is an inflammation of the kidney. It can be a bacterial infection (acute) or related to other factors (chronic).

PATHOPHYSIOLOGY
In chronic conditions, the infection migrates from the lower urinary tract to the kidney. Most acute infections are caused by E. coli, Proteus, or Klebsiella.

ASSOCIATED MEDICAL CONDITIONS
- Vesicoureteral reflex

ASSESSMENT
- Signs and symptoms of lower urinary tract infection
- C & S of urine
- Chills
- Headache
- Flank pain
- Hypertension (chronic pyelonephritis)
- Frequency, burning on urination
- Low-grade fever
- Malaise
- Hematuria
- Dysuria
- Excessive thirst

CLIENT NEED:
Physiological integrity

NURSING INTERVENTIONS
- Force fluids, 3L/day
- Administer antibiotics

PATIENT TEACHING
- Instruct female patient to wipe front to back
- The purpose of long-term, regular antibiotic therapy
- Instruct female patient to urinate after intercourse
- Encourage intake 3L/day, especially cranberry juice

- Recognize signs/symptoms of infection

ASSOCIATED NURSING DIAGNOSES
- Fatigue
- Knowledge deficit
- Physical mobility, impaired
- Urinary retention
- Infection, high risk for
- Pain
- Skin integrity, impaired
- Urinary elimination, altered

STUDY QUESTION

■ A urine C&S is obtained in the patient with pyelonephritis. This test is important because the physician will utilize it in:
1. Making the diagnosis
2. Determining length of treatment
3. Prescribing medication of choice
4. Prescribing pain medications

Answer: 3. Prescribing medication of choice

Rationale: The cultural and sensitivity targets the causative organism and, therefore, the antimicrobial agents to kill the pathogen.

Nursing process: Intervention

Client need: Physiological integrity

> Clinical skill level: 3

RENAL CALCULI

DEFINITION
Renal calculi (or stones) are a soft tissue calcification that originates in the kidney and are carried by the urine into the collecting system, causing severe pain and urinary obstruction.

PATHOPHYSIOLOGY
Stones are formed from excess crystals in the urine. Different conditions can produce crystals, such as gout, calcium, or urinary tract infection.

ASSESSMENT
- Sharp severe flank and back pain
- Nausea and vomiting
- Pallor
- Chills
- Decreasing urinary output
- RUB to determine location of stone
- Diaphoresis
- Urinary frequency
- Dysuria
- Abdominal cramping associated with gross hematuria

CLIENT NEED
Physiological integrity

NURSING INTERVENTIONS
- Administer pain medications, usually Demoral IM
- Strict I & O
- Avoid diet high in purine:
  - Red meats
  - Bouillon
  - Sardines
  - Meat extracts
- Strain all urine
- Collect mid-stream urine
- Restrict dairy products; particularly Vitamin D

- Broths, gravy, consommé
- Yeast
- Sweetbreads
• Encourage alkaline ash diet:
  - Legumes
  - Green vegetables
  - Fruits (except prunes, cranberries)
  - Halibut
  - Salmon

PATIENT TEACHING

- Encourage fluid intake (3-4L/day)
- Promptly report any signs of urinary tract infection
- Measure I&O
- Instruct that Vitamin D enhances calcium absorption and should be decreased when possible.

ASSOCIATED NURSING DIAGNOSES

- Pain
- Coping, ineffective individual
- Urinary retention
- Activity intolerance
- Nutrition, less than body requirements, altered
- Urinary elimination, altered

STUDY QUESTIONS

■ The patient who is prone to urinary stones is put on an alkaline ash diet. The nurse recommends all fruits except:
1. Oranges and bananas
2. Oranges and cranberries
3. Apples and plums
4. Cranberries and prunes

Answer: 4. Cranberries and prunes

Rationale: Cranberries, prunes and plums are exceptions to the alkaline ash diet because they tend to make urine more acidic.

Nursing Process: Intervention

Client Need: Physiological integrity

Clinical skill level: 3

■ The patient who has recurrent UTI is prescribed an acid ash diet in an attempt to decrease the formation of renal stones. Dietary selections include:
1. Eggs, meat, cereals
2. Legumes and ham
3. Milk and prunes
4. All fruit except cranberries

Answer: 1. Eggs, meat, cereals

Rationale: In addition, the acid ash diet also includes prunes, cranberries, asparagus, tomatoes and corn.

Nursing process: Intervention

Client need: Physiological integrity

Clinical skill level: 3

RENAL FAILURE

DEFINITION
Renal failure is the loss of kidney function. It may be either acute (in which the kidneys stop functioning abruptly), or chronic (in which the renal tissue progressively stops functioning). In either case, the healthy renal tissue which is still functioning can no longer handle the demands of the body, and, eventually, shut down occurs.

PATHOPHYSIOLOGY
The mechanisms that lead to the renal failure can be many and complex. Primarily, failure is related to a pathological process that causes renal ischemia or to renal injury.

Stages of renal failure:
- Oliguric phase:
  - Initial clinical manifestations of failure being. Oliguria is the cardinal sign. This stage may begin as soon as 24 hours after the cause initiates failure and last up to 2 weeks.
- Diuretic phase
  - Output increases, perhaps up to 5L/day, for the duration of the phase, which may be up to 3 weeks.
- Recovery phase:
  - Major recovery within 2 weeks but may continue up to a year.

ASSOCIATED MEDICAL CONDITIONS
- Burns
- Anaphylaxis
- Crushing injuries
- Medications, especially aminoglycosides
- Myocardial infarction
- Hemorrhage
- Glomerulonephritis
- Pyelonephritis

ASSESSMENT
- Azotemia
- Oliguria (output > 400 ml/day)
- Uremia
- Edema, obvious in bounding neck veins

- Elevated BUN
- Elevated potassium
- Hypertension
- Elevated creatinine
- Hematuria

CLIENT NEED
Physiological integrity

NURSING INTERVENTIONS
- Administer diuretic therapy, such as furosemide (Lasix) or Mannitol.
- Monitor sodium and potassium levels
- Monitor strict I&O
- Be alert for fluid and electrolyte imbalances, especially metabolic acidosis
- Monitor BUN, creatinine levels

PATIENT TEACHING
- Teach strict I&O
- Teach to recognize each of the three phases of renal failure
- Be alert for urinary retention

ASSOCIATED NURSING DIAGNOSES
- Anxiety
- Fear
- Tissue perfusion, altered, renal
- Fatigue
- Pain, chronic
- Urinary retention

STUDY QUESTIONS

■ The ICU nurse observes the patient in renal failure for ECG changes, Kussmaul breathing, and decreased LOC. This assessment is monitoring for:
1. Response to dialysis
2. Metabolic alkalosis
3. Electrolyte imbalance
4. Cardiac complications

Answer: 3. Electrolyte imbalance

Rationale: Another complication of renal failure is electrolyte imbalance, particularly hyperkalemia because it is the most life-threatening. Hyperkalemia can cause dysrhythmias that lead to cardiac arrest.

Nursing process: Assessment

Client need: Physiological integrity

Clinical skill level: 3

■ A patient in renal failure has a decreased ability to excrete protein wastes. Which lab test reflects this condition?
1. A high BUN
2. A drop in BUN
3. High creatinine levels
4. High SGOT level

Answer: 1. A high BUN

Rationale: BUN measures the nitrogen factor in urea, which is the end product of protein metabolism. BUN is an indicator of the kidney's capacity to excrete waste.

Nursing process: Evaluation

Client need: Physiological integrity

Clinical skill level: 2

URINARY TRACT INFECTION

DEFINITION
The second most common bacterial disease, urinary tract infections may appear as a number of disorders. The infections occur as a result of microbial invasion of the urinary tract tissues, primarily by Escherichia coli. UTI's occur more frequently in women than in men and are linked to sexual activity and pregnancy.

PATHOPHYSIOLOGY
Although the bladder is resistant to infection, an indwelling catheter, calculus, tumor or parasites can damage the mucosal lining of the bladder, making possible the invasion of bacterial organisms. Additionally, urine stasis contributes to bacterial growth. Other sources of infection may include the patient's own colon. Untreated infections may become recurrent.

MOST COMMON MEDICAL CONDITIONS
- Pyelonephritis

ASSESSMENT
- Foul-smelling urine
- Suprapubic pain
- Burning on urination
- Malaise
- Fever
- Vomiting
- Low back pain
- Hematuria
- Dysuria
- Chills
- Nausea

CLIENT NEED
Physiological integrity

NURSING INTERVENTIONS
- Administer antimicrobials
- Administer antibiotics (ampicillin, amoxicillin)

- Acid ash diet for patients with recurrent infections
- Administer sulfonamides
- Encourage fluid intake of 3000 ml/day (especially cranberry juice)

PATIENT TEACHING
- Void after sexual intercourse
- Avoid bubble baths and perfumed soap
- Avoid tight clothing which traps heat in perineal area
- Drink 3000 ml of water per day

ASSOCIATED NURSING DIAGNOSES
- Anxiety
- Fatigue
- Physical mobility, impaired
- Urinary retention
- Pain
- Infection, high risk for
- Nutrition: less than body requirements, altered
- Urinary elimination, altered

STUDY QUESTIONS

■ Post-operatively a patient voids 50 ml of clear yellow urine three times, but continues to complain that the bladder does not feel empty. The nurse evaluates this symptom as:
1. Hypodiasis
2. Enuresis
3. Retention with overflow
4. Stress incontinence

Answer: 3. Retention with overflow

Rationale: Urinary retention with overflow following an operation is believed to be caused by a spasm of the bladder sphincter.

Nursing process: Evaluation

Client need: Physiological integrity

Clinical skill level: 2

■ The cardinal symptom of a bladder infection is:
1. Chill
2. Dysuria
3. Back pain
4. Stress incontinence

Answer: 2. Dysuria

Rationale: Dysuria means difficulty voiding. Included among the symptoms are burning pain, hesitancy and frequency.

Nursing process: Assessment

Client need: Physiological integrity

Clinical skill level: 2

■ The doctor orders a clean, voided specimen. What does the nurse instruct the patient to do when obtaining this specimen?
1. Collect the first urine voided
2. Collect urine during midstream voiding
3. Sterilize the meatus as much as possible
4. Void completely into a clean urine cup

Answer: 2. Collect urine during midstream voiding

Rationale: A midstream specimen does not contain the bacteria usually found around the urethral meatus because the first-voided urine will help wash it away.

Nursing process: Intervention

Client need: Physiological integrity

Clinical skill level: 2

■ In planning care, the nurse is aware that the greatest risk of urinary catheterization is:
1. Bladder irritation
2. Meatal swelling
3. Bladder puncture
4. Urinary tract infection

Answer: 4. Urinary tract infection

Rationale: UTIs occur frequently due to the placement of the catheter, as it provides a direct tract for bacteria to traverse. The primary cause of UTI is *E. Coli* from fecal material.

Nursing process: Assessment

Client need: Health promotion and maintenance

Clinical skill level: 2

■ In guarding against urinary tract infection, which nursing intervention is best?
1. Frequent ambulation, ROM
2. Forcing fluids
3. Emptying bladder every 8 hours
4. Emptying catheter bag frequently

Answer: 2. Forcing fluids

Rationale: Encouraging fluids will force the patient to urinate more often, flushing bacteria out of the urinary tract.

Nursing process: Intervention

Client need: Physiological integrity

Clinical skill level: 2

General Study Questions

■ The average adult excretes how much urine in a usual 24-hour period?
1. 100-200 cc
2. 500-700 cc
3. 700-900 cc
4. 1200-1800 cc

Answer: 4. 1200-1800 cc
Rationale: The normal adult produces approximately 60 cc to 70 cc of urine per hour.
Nursing process: Outcome criteria
Client need: Physiological integrity

Clinical skill level: 2

■ Which record of urinary output is minimally acceptable, but would alert the nurse to problems?
1. Less than 30 cc/hour
2. Less than 60 cc/hour
3. Less than 90 cc/hour
4. Less than 120 cc/hour

Answer: 1. Less than 30 cc/hour
Rationale: The minimum urine output is 30 cc/hour.
Nursing process: Assessment
Client need: Physiological integrity

Clinical skill level: 2

■ How much urine can the bladder normally hold?
   1. 100 cc
   2. 200 cc
   3. 400 cc
   4. 600 cc

   Answer: 4. 600 cc

   Rationale: The receptors in the bladder usually begin signaling urination is necessary at about 600 cc.

   Nursing process: Assessment

   Client need: Physiological integrity

   Clinical skill level: 1

■ A patient's Foley catheter is to be DC'd in the a.m. After explaining the procedure, the next thing the nurse should do before removing the catheter is:
   1. Deflate the balloon
   2. Gently remove the catheter
   3. Place a towel under the buttocks
   4. Empty urine from the bag

   Answer: 1. Deflate the balloon

   Rationale: The balloon must be deflated first to prevent tissue damage during the removal of the catheter.

   Nursing process: Intervention

   Client need: Physiological integrity

   Clinical skill level: 2

■ The physician orders a urine specimen to test for glucose and ketones. The nurse obtains which specimen?
1. Sterile
2. Midstream
3. Double-voided
4. Clean single-voided

Answer: 3. Double-voided

Rationale: Double-voided means to throw away the first specimen and to run the test on the second specimen. This method is believed to provide a more accurate reflection of the urine glucose.

Nursing process: Intervention

Client need: Physiological integrity

Clinical skill level: 2

■ A male patient, 62, had surgery for inguinal hernia repair 8 hours ago. He has not voided. What nursing intervention can help him void?
1. Assist him to stand at the bedside
2. Place his hands in warm water
3. Pour cool water over his perineum
4. Turn the water faucet on and let it run

Answer: 1. Assist him to stand at the bedside

Rationale: Standing is a natural position for males and will help to initiate micturition.

Nursing process: Intervention

Client need: Physiological integrity

Clinical skill level: 2

- A patient has an indwelling catheter. How would the nurse obtain a sterile urine specimen?
  1. Disconnect catheter from the tubing
  2. Empty it from the drainage bag
  3. Empty it from the urometer
  4. Use a sterile needle to withdraw it from the catheter port

  Answer: 4. Use a sterile needle to withdraw it from the catheter port

  Rationale: The only way that the urine will not be further contaminated is by using a sterile needle and injecting the specimen into a sterile container.

  Nursing process: Intervention

  Client need: Safe, effective care environment

  Clinical skill level: 2

- During a 24-hour urine collection, what instructions should be given regarding the first and last specimen?
  1. Both specimens should be discarded
  2. Both specimens should be sent to lab
  3. Discard first specimen, send last specimen to lab
  4. Send first specimen to lab, discard last specimen

  Answer: 3. Discard first specimen, send last specimen to lab

  Rationale: The first urine specimen collected must be discarded. The 24-hour collection period begins and ends when the bladder is completely empty.

  Nursing process: Intervention

  Client need: Health promotion and maintenance

  Clinical skill level: 2

- A priority nursing intervention following removal of an indwelling catheter is:
  1. Ambulation
  2. Restrict fluids
  3. Force fluids
  4. Pain management

  Answer: 3. Force fluids

  Rationale: High fluid intake is recommended so the bladder will begin to empty frequently, avoiding build-up of bacteria. Another reason is to "retrain" the bladder as it is elastic and tends to get "lazy" muscle tone when not filled and emptied often.

  Nursing process: Intervention

  Client need: Health promotion and maintenance

  Clinical skill level: 2

- The nurse is evaluating a battery of pre-operative tests. The serum creatinine level reflects:
  1. Cardiac function
  2. Endocrine function
  3. Pulmonary function
  4. Renal function

  Answer: 4. Renal function

  Rationale: Creatinine a waste product of muscle that is excreted through glomerular filtration. The amount of creatinine filter equals the amount in urine because it is not reabsorbed by the renal tubules. Because of this it is the most accurate measure of renal function.

  Nursing process: Assessment

  Client need: Physiological integrity

  Clinical skill level: 3

■ Which finding is prominent in the urine of a patient with acute glomerulonephritis?
1. White cells
2. Platelets
3. Protein
4. Calculi

Answer: 3. Protein

Rationale: The urine is scanty and bloody with a large amount of protein.

Nursing process: Assessment

Client need: Physiological integrity

Clinical skill level: 3

■ In planning care of the hospitalized patient with a urinary calculi, a priority is placed on:
1. Catheter care
2. Strict bed rest
3. Water restriction
4. Straining of urine

Answer: 4. Straining of urine

Rationale: If the patient passes the stone, the only way to know is to strain the urine.

Nursing process: Assessment

Client need: Physiological integrity

Clinical skill level: 2

■ In caring for the patient in acute renal failure, the nurse is aware that a major complication is:
1. Hypertension
2. Hypocalcemia
3. Hyperkalemia
4. Hypokalemia

Answer: 3. Hyperkalemia

Rationale: As function is compromised, the kidneys are unable to excrete potassium. In addition, protein catabolism causes an increase in potassium in the blood. The complication of hyperkalemia is cardiac dysrythmias.

Nursing process:

Client need: Physiological integrity

Clinical skill level: 3

■ The nurse is planning discharge for the patient who recently underwent a renal transplant. She stresses the importance of measuring urine output and taking temperature and blood pressure. These readings are important because they could signal:
1. Renal failure
2. Heart failure
3. Hypovolemic shock
4. A rejection episode

Answer: 4. A rejection episode

Rationale: Fever, decreased output and increasing blood pressure are signs of rejection and must be reported to the physician immediately.

Nursing process: Evaluation

Client need: Physiological integrity

Clinical skill level: 4

■ A patient is scheduled for peritoneal dialysis. What important nursing intervention must be taken before dialysis is initiated?
1. Administer pain medication
2. Place patient in high-Fowler's
3. Weigh the patient
4. Instruct on complications

Answer: 3. Weigh the patient

Rationale: The best way for the nurse to assess if the patient is retaining fluid is by weighing before and after the procedure.

Nursing process: Evaluation

Client need: Physiological integrity

Clinical skill level: 3

■ The physician orders barium studies and an intravenous pyelogram. Which should the nurse schedule first?
1. The barium studies
2. The intravenous pyelogram
3. It doesn't make any difference
4. They should be performed at the same time

Answer: 2. The intravenous pyelogram

Rationale: Since residual barium may obscure organs, the studies using iodine contrast medium should be scheduled first.

Nursing process: Intervention

Client need: Physiological integrity

Clinical skill level: 3

- The nurse is monitoring the patient on hemodialysis. The signs and symptoms of complications are:
    1. Tetany, weakness, chest pain, dysrhythmias
    2. Tachycardia, hypotension, headache
    3. Anasarca, headache, malaise
    4. Respiratory distress, generalized weakness

    Answer: 1. Tetany, weakness, chest pain, dysrhythmias
    Rationale: Complications associated with dialysis are often caused by drop in potassium levels. this causes tetany, muscle weakness, and dysrhythmias. Shifts in fluid volume will cause the chest pain.
    Nursing process: Evaluation
    Client need: Physiological integrity

    Clinical skill level: 3

- A patient is diagnosed with glomerulonephritis. The nurse should be alert for which common complications?
    1. High fever and edema
    2. Frequent colds and fever
    3. Urinary tract infections
    4. Hypertension and facial edema

    Answer: 4. Hypertension and facial edema
    Rationale: The kidneys are large and swollen due to an inflammatory reaction in the kidneys. The kidneys become congested, unable to filter fluids, leading to hypertension and edema.
    Nursing process: Assessment
    Client need: Physiological integrity

    Clinical skill level: 2

■ What common complications of glomerulonephritis tend to recur frequently?
1. Fever and edema
2. Frequent colds and fever
3. Urinary tract infections
4. Hypertension and edema

Answer: 4. Hypertension and edema.

Rationale: Hypertension and edema, along with headaches and oliguria, are common complications of this disease.

Nursing process: Evaluation

Client need: Physiological integrity

Clinical skill level: 3

■ The nurse assesses the renal patient's mental status. If there is a problem, what condition is most likely to be assessed?
1. Aggression
2. Delirium
3. Confusion
4. Intense anger

Answer: 3. Confusion

Rationale: In renal disease, urea is not being filtered by the kidneys and is building up in the blood, resulting in toxicity to brain tissue, causing confusion.

Nursing process: Assessment

Client need: Physiological integrity

Clinical skill level: 4

UNIT 9
GASTROINTESTINAL SYSTEM

- Peptic Ulcers
- Hepatitis A
- Hepatitis B
- Cirrhosis of the Liver

PEPTIC ULCERS

DEFINITION
A peptic ulcer is a break in the esophageal, gastric, or duodenal mucosa. Peptic ulcers may occur in any part of the gastrointestinal tract which comes in contact with gastric juices. Roughly 10% of American men and 4% of women will develop duodenal ulcers, which comprise about 80% of peptic ulcers.

PATHOPHYSIOLOGY
Endocrine hormones and cortisone change the structure of the esophageal, gastric and duodenal mucosa and the amount of mucus produced. Adrenocorticosteroids make the mucus more susceptible to injury and may reduce the renewal of mucosal cells. Stress can also increase gastric secretion. When stress occurs, blood vessels constrict, and the mucosa becomes vulnerable to trauma. Once the mucosal barrier has been damaged, hydrochloric acid enters and further damages the tissue. The mucosa releases histamine which causes vasodilation and makes the capillaries permeable. The histamine leads to additional secretion of acid and pepsin.

NURSING ASSESSMENT
- Aching, burning pain
- Bleeding
- Occult bleeding
- Nausea and vomiting
- Massive hemorrhage

CLIENT NEED
Physiological integrity

NURSING INTERVENTIONS
- Administer ranitidine hydrochloride to block action of H_2 receptors to reduce gastric secretion
- Administer Sucralfate to form protective coat that prevents digestive action of acid and pepsin

- Administer anticholinergics
- Carefully monitor for drug interactions when taking Tagamet
- Administer cimetidine (Tagamet) for short-term therapy

PATIENT TEACHING
- Observe medication schedule
- Advise no smoking with cimetidine (Tagamet) or Zantac
- Find ways of dealing with stressors
- Eat nutritionally balanced diet
- Use acetaminophen instead of aspirin (aspirin is ulcerogenic)
- Advise no aspirin or alcohol intake when taking Tagamet or Zantac (may increase GI irritation)

ASSOCIATED NURSING DIAGNOSES
- Knowledge deficit
- Pain, chronic
- Injury, high risk for
- Nutrition: less than body requirements, altered
- Noncompliance
- Health-seeking behaviors

STUDY QUESTIONS

■ In explaining how the diagnosis of peptic ulcer is made, the nurse states the best diagnostic method is:
  1. Barium swallow
  2. Barium enema
  3. Endoscopy
  4. Stool specimen

  Answer: 3. Endoscopy
  Rationale: Endoscopic therapy is also used to control bleeding if the patient begins to hemorrhage.
  Nursing process: Intervention
  Client need: Physiological integrity

  Clinical skill level: 2

■ A patient with a peptic ulcer experiences severe pain in the abdomen. The abdomen is extremely rigid and tender. This patient shows early signs of shock with a dropping blood pressure. The nurse suspects:
1. Perforation
2. More than an ulcer
3. Pyloric obstruction
4. Nothing abnormal

Answer: 1. Perforation

Rationale: The sharp pain and sudden drop in BP is indicative of internal hemorrhage.

Nursing process: Assessment

Client need: Physiological integrity

Clinical skill level: 3

■ The patient diagnosed with a peptic ulcer is prescribed Tagamet (cimetidine). The nurse instructs the patient that this medication will:
1. Cause weight gain
2. Cause bloody stools
3. Cause palpitations
4. Facilitate healing

Answer: 4. Facilitate healing

Rationale: Tagamet is an H2 antagonist that reduces gastric secretions, particularly histamine, and reduces irritation.

Nursing process: Intervention

Client need: Physiological integrity

Clinical skill level: 2

- The patient diagnosed with peptic ulcers is requesting aspirin for his headache. Patient teaching focuses on the fact that he should avoid taking aspirin because this drug may:
    1. Cause diarrhea
    2. Cause nausea
    3. Cause bleeding
    4. Not relieve the pain

    Answer: 3. Cause bleeding

    Rationale: A major complication of gastric ulcers is GI bleeding, and aspirin decreases clotting time.

    Nursing process: Intervention

    Client need: Physiological integrity

    Clinical skill level: 2

- The patient is scheduled for an upper GI series. Patient teaching includes caution against smoking. The rationale for this is because smoking:
    1. Can stimulate gastric motility
    2. Causes contrast medium to dissolve
    3. Causes esophageal varices
    4. Decreases absorption of the dye

    Answer: 1. Can stimulate gastric motility

    Rationale: Nicotine stimulates the GI tract by increasing the tone and motor activity of GI tract smooth muscle.

    Nursing process: Intervention

    Client need: Physiological integrity

    Clinical skill level: 2

■ A patient is hospitalized with a peptic ulcer after suddenly vomiting 500 ml of blood. The priority nursing intervention is:
1. Administration of normal saline IV
2. Removal of the nasogastric tube
3. Notifying the operating room
4. Reinserting nasogastric tube stat

Answer: 1. Administration of normal saline IV

Rationale: The priority is to maintain circulating volume and prevent hypovolemia. Normal saline will be administered.

Nursing process: Intervention

Client need: Physiological integrity

Clinical skill level: 2

CIRRHOSIS OF THE LIVER

DEFINITION
Cirrhosis means scarring of the liver.

PATHOPHYSIOLOGY
- There are three causes of cirrhosis:
  - Alcoholism,
  - Scarring from hepatitis, and
  - Scarring that results from chronic biliary obstruction or inflammation.

ASSOCIATED MEDICAL CONDITIONS
- Laennec's cirrhosis (associated with alcoholism)
- Ascites

ASSESSMENT
- Palpation of liver
- Indigestion
- Diarrhea
- Hemorrhoids
- Dullness upon percussion of abdomen
- Spider telangiectases, especially on face
- Abdominal pain
- Constipation
- Weight loss
- Ascites
- Fluid wave upon percussion of abdomen

Late signs:
- Edema
- Chronic gastritis
- Anemia
- Decreasing cognitive ability

CLIENT NEED
Physiological integrity

NURSING INTERVENTIONS

- Administer antacids
- Administer diuretics (if ascites present)
- Patterns of alcohol use
- Administer O_2
- Strict I&O
- Promote optimal nutrition
- Avoid alcohol
- Encourage adequate rest
- Daily weight

PATIENT TEACHING

- Teach damaging effects of alcohol
- Importance of low salt diet
- Importance of good nutrition, especially high protein, high calorie
- Report any weight gain for physician
- Importance of high fiber diet

ASSOCIATED NURSING DIAGNOSES

- Anxiety
- Constipation
- Fear
- Fluid volume excess
- Pain, chronic
- Nutrition: less than body requirements, altered
- Activity intolerance
- Fatigue
- Hopelessness
- Physical mobility, impaired
- Skin integrity, impaired

STUDY QUESTIONS

■ Even though the cirrhosis patient has ascites, the nurse should encourage:
   1. Regular diet
   2. Fiber restriction
   3. Fluid intake
   4. Moderate alcohol intake

Answer: 3. Fluid intake

Rationale: Adequate fluid intake is required because fever and increased metabolic rate causes loss of fluid through perspiration and evaporation.

Nursing process: Intervention

Client need: Physiological integrity

Clinical skill level: 4

■ In patient teaching the cirrhosis patient about his diet, which nutrient should the nurse emphasize must comprise the bulk of the diet?
   1. Complex carbohydrates
   2. Complete protein
   3. Incomplete protein
   4. Water and other liquids

Answer: 1. Complex carbohydrates

Rationale: Complex carbohydrates are required for energy for this patient who is fatigued and may be running a fever. Proteins will be restricted because the impaired liver can metabolize only small amounts of protein at a time.

Nursing process: Intervention

Client need: Physiological integrity

Clinical skill level: 4

■ The patient asks the nurse, "Why do I have to be on a low-salt diet? I don't have a heart problem." The nurse answers that a low-salt diet helps to prevent:
1. Pain
2. Infection
3. Fever
4. Edema

Answer: 4. Edema

Rationale: Sodium enhances the fluid retention that is already prominent in the patient with cirrhosis.

Nursing process: Intervention

Client need: Physiological integrity

Clinical skill level: 4

HEPATITIS A

DEFINITION
Hepatitis A is an inflammation of the liver caused by the RNA virus. The liver becomes tender and jaundice sets in. The virus can be found in the stool two or more weeks before symptoms appear and three to four week before the onset of jaundice.

PATHOPHYSIOLOGY
Hepatitis A causes widespread inflammation of the liver tissue and damages liver cells through hepatic cell degeneration. Kupffer cells proliferate and become enlarged and bile flow may be interrupted due to inflammation of the periportal areas. Cholestasis may also occur.

ASSESSMENT
Preicteric phase:
- Anorexia
- Nausea
- Malaise
- Low grade fever
- Rash
- Abdominal discomfort
- Headache

Icteric phase:
- Jaundice
- Fatigue
- Pruritus

CLIENT NEED
Physiological integrity

NURSING INTERVENTIONS
- Administer immunoglobin
- Enteric precautions
- Small, frequent meals to ensure adequate nutrition and prevent nausea
- Isolation precautions for 1 week after onset of jaundice
- Scheduled rest periods

PATIENT TEACHING

- Avoid alcohol and sedatives
- Avoid raw shellfish
- Avoid sexual activity until symptoms abate
- Importance of good personal hygiene (Hepatitis A is transmitted primarily through the fecal/oral route)

ASSOCIATED NURSING DIAGNOSES

- Activity intolerance
- Diarrhea
- Pain
- Anxiety
- Fatigue
- Nutrition: less than body requirements, altered

STUDY QUESTIONS

■ In assessing the patient with Hepatitis A, the nurse recognizes that the first signs and symptoms are this disease are:
1. High fever and vomiting
2. Petechiae and hepatomegaly
3. Jaundice and dark urine
4. Constipation alternating with diarrhea

Answer: 1. High fever and vomiting

Rationale: This highly infectious process starts with fever and vomiting. Other signs are anorexia associated with nausea and chills.

Nursing process: Assessment

Client need: Physiological integrity

Clinical skill level: 3

- Isolation is ordered for the patient with Hepatitis A. The nurse prepares to implement:
    1. Universal precautions
    2. Respiratory isolation
    3. Enteric precautions
    4. Strict isolation

    Answer: 3. Enteric precautions

    Rationale: The Hepatitis A virus lives in the feces and is transmitted via fecal contamination by the infected person. Enteric precautions reduce the risk of contact with the infective agent.

    Nursing process: Intervention

    Client need: Physiological integrity

    Clinical skill level: 3

- During the course of treatment the nurse will pay particular attention to which of the following tests results?
    1. WBCs
    2. BUN
    3. Creatinine clearance
    4. Serum transaminase

    Answer: 4. Serum transaminase

    Rationale: High elevations of serum transaminase occur as a result of hepatocellular inflammation. The level begins to drop quickly once recovery occurs.

    Nursing process: Evaluation

    Client need: Physiological integrity

    Clinical skill level: 4

HEPATITIS B

DEFINITION
An inflammation of the liver caused by a blood-borne pathogen and can be spread by several routes, including sexual contact, shared needles, needlesticks, blood transfusions, or contaminated body fluids.

PATHOPHYSIOLOGY
The incubation period is long, 45-160 days. Although the actual factors involved in the liver damage are not yet clear, the disease is characterized by the following changes in the liver:
- Necrosis of liver cells
- Inflammation by leukocytes
- Regeneration of liver tissue

ASSOCIATED MEDICAL CONDITIONS
- Chronic active hepatitis
- Chronic persistent hepatitis
- Postnecrotic cirrhosis

ASSESSMENT
- Degree of exposure in healthcare workplace
- Fatigue
- Enlarged liver
- Abnormal liver function tests
- Diminished appetite/anorexia
- Abdominal pain
- Jaundice
- Tobacco-colored urine

CLIENT NEED
Physiological integrity

NURSING INTERVENTIONS

- Maintain nutritional status with offerings of small, frequent, high caloric meals/snacks
- Maintain universal precautions
- Monitor fluid volume status
- Administer Hepatitis B vaccine, preexposure (preferably) or postexposure. This consists of three IM injections, with the second and third injections given at 1 and 6 months.
- Provide for optimal periods of rest with activity restriction

MEDICAL INTERVENTIONS

- Microbiologic studies to detect disease
- Mild antiemetic to control nausea/anorexia

PATIENT TEACHING

- Teach the need for rest and optimal nutrition
- Vaccine is expensive, but all three injections must be administered for immunization to be effective
- Instruct not to ever give blood for transfusions
- Instruct regarding signs and symptoms of liver failure

ASSOCIATED NURSING DIAGNOSES

- Activity intolerance, high risk for
- Infection, high risk for
- Pain
- Nutrition, less than body requirements, altered
- Fatigue
- Role performance, altered

STUDY QUESTIONS

■ In taking a patient history, the patient who is suspected of being HBV positive has difficulty pinpointing when he may have been exposed. This is primarily because Hepatitis B:
1. Is very difficult to contact
2. Has a long incubation period
3. Has a very short incubation period
4. Has very subtle signs and symptoms

Answer: 2. Has a long incubation period
Rationale: The incubation period for Hepatitis B is 45-160 days. A person who is not aware of immediate potential exposure to this blood-borne pathogen may not remember when it occurred. Exposure occurs most commonly through needlesticks and sexual contact.
Nursing process: Assessment
Client need: Physiological integrity

Clinical skill level: 3

■ In discharge teaching, the nurse emphasizes to the patient diagnosed with Hepatitis B:
1. Abstain from sex for 6 weeks
2. Do not eat uncooked shellfish
3. Never donate blood for transfusion
4. Should avoid any immunizations

Answer: 3. Never donate blood for transfusion
Rationale: HBV is blood-borne pathogen that is transmitted via blood transfusions and a person who has been diagnosed should never donate blood.
Nursing process: Intervention
Client need: Physiological integrity

Clinical skill level: 3

GENERAL STUDY QUESTIONS

■ The patient has just had a liver biopsy. The patient should be positioned:
1. In a side-lying position
2. In a supine position
3. In a prone position
4. Sitting up leaning toward the left

Answer: 1. In a side-lying position

Rationale: Since the liver is highly vascular, hemorrhage is a risk following biopsy. The pressure created in the lateral position will decrease the chance of bleeding.

Nursing process: Intervention

Client need: Physiological integrity

Clinical skill level: 2

■ A 50-year-old mother of four is suffering acute cholecystitis with jaundice. the jaundice would be categorized as:
1. Hemolytic jaundice
2. Obstructive jaundice
3. Hepatocellular
4. Hepatic syndrome

Answer: 2. Obstructive jaundice

Rationale: Obstructive jaundice is caused by obstructed bile flow. The bile backs up in the liver and causes bilirubin to be reabsorbed into the blood.

Nursing process: Evaluation

Client need: Physiological integrity

Clinical skill level: 2

- The cardinal sign of an impaction is:
    1. Small amount of hard stool
    2. Frequent passage of liquid stool
    3. Nausea and vomiting
    4. Chronic constipation

    Answer: 2. Frequent passage of liquid stool
    Rationale: Watery stool that is forced out of the rectum around impacted feces is a sign of impaction as is constipation.
    Nursing process: Assessment
    Client need: Physiological integrity

    Clinical skill level: 1

- The nurse observes that the patient with an NG tube is experiencing significant coughing and gagging. A priority assessment should be:
    1. Check cough medication
    2. Check tube placement
    3. Check aspirated contents
    4. Check for bleeding from tube

    Answer: 2. Check tube placement
    Rationale: Coughing and gagging can cause the tube to slip out of place, and placement should be checked each time liquid is administered.
    Nursing Process: Assessment
    Client need: Safe, effective care environment

    Clinical skill level: 3

- Fifteen minutes after insertion of an NG tube, the nurse assesses that the patient is experiencing bradycardia. This new sign is recognized as a potential complication because it is indicative of:
  1. Vagal stimulation
  2. Impending MI
  3. Hypovolemic shock
  4. Paralytic ileus

  Answer: 1. Vagal stimulation

  Rationale: If the patient experiences bradycardia, the tube should be withdrawn and the physician notified. Vagal stimulation may set off cardiac dysrhythmias and bradycardia is an early sign.

  Nursing process: Evaluation

  Client Need: Physiological integrity

  > Clinical skill level: 3

- The nurse asks the patient to sit in a high-Fowler's position for the insertion of a nasogastric tube. In addition to facilitating the insertion of the tube, another important reason for this position is that it:
  1. Forces patient to assist with insertion
  2. Prevents aspiration should vomiting occur
  3. Is the only way the tube can be inserted
  4. Is the only way to test for placement

  Answer: 2. Prevents aspiration should vomiting occur

  Rationale: There is a chance the patient may gag and vomit during insertion of the NG tube. The vomitus should be cleared expediently in order to prevent aspiration.

  Nursing process: Intervention

  Client need: Safe, effective care environment

  > Clinical skill level: 2

- Which of the following methods should the nurse use to determine the correct distance to insert a nasogastric tube?
    1. Center of forehead to tip of nose to end of sternum
    2. Tip of nose to tip of earlobe to end of sternum
    3. Lips to tip of ear to just below the umbilicus
    4. Top of ear to midway between end of sternum and umbilicus

    Answer: 2. Tip of nose to tip of earlobe to end of sternum
    Rationale: The distance measured is the approximate distance from the nose into the stomach.
    Nursing process: Intervention
    Client need: Physiological integrity

    Clinical skill level: 2

- What is the most accurate method of determining that a nasogastric tube is in the stomach?
    1. Attach a syringe; aspirate gastric contents
    2. Hold it under water; listen for air flow with a stethoscope
    3. Insert 5 ml water; listen for air flow with a stethoscope
    4. Insert 2 ml water; listen for gurgling with stethoscope

    Answer: 1. Attach a syringe; aspirate gastric contents
    Rationale: Stomach contents can be aspirated only if the tube has entered the stomach.
    Nursing process: Intervention
    Client need: Physiological integrity

    Clinical skill level: 2

■ Acute pancreatitis is best diagnosed by which of the following studies?
1. Serum amylase level
2. Serum glucose level
3. Serum bilirubin level
4. White blood cell

Answer: 1. Serum amylase level

Rationale: Serum amylase is elevated in pancreatitis because

Nursing process: Evaluation

Client need: Physiological integrity

Clinical skill level: 3

■ A patient is recovering from an attack of acute pancreatitis. The NG tube has been removed. Which meal is the best choice for lunch?
1. A fruit salad plate
2. An egg salad plate
3. A cheeseburger
4. A tuna salad sandwich

Answer: 1. A fruit salad plate

Rationale: A well-balanced, low-fat diet as well as a diet high in protein and carbohydrates that is supplemented by vitamin replacement encourages hepatic regeneration. Small frequent meals are tolerated better than large ones.

Nursing process: Intervention

Client need: Physiological integrity

Clinical skill level: 3

■ A patient undergoes a total gastrectomy. Following gastric surgery the patient complains of weakness and palpitations. Teaching includes the requirement of vitamin B_{12} injections for life because:
1. The oral form is not available
2. Lack of intrinsic factor
3. The body cannot absorb it
4. The gastric process requires more of it

Answer: 2. Lack of intrinsic factor

Rationale: The intrinsic factor required for B_{12} absorption is removed in a gastrectomy.

Nursing process: Evaluation

Client need: Physiological integrity

Clinical skill level: 3

■ An assessment method to evaluate care of the patient with diarrhea is to:
1. Measure abdominal girth
2. Palpate the abdomen
3. Auscultate bowel sounds
4. Percuss over lower quadrant

Answer: 3. Auscultate bowel sounds

Rationale: Bowel sounds are usually growling and loud when a patient is having diarrhea. Less aggressive sounds will indicate the bowel is settling down and the diarrhea abating.

Nursing process: Evaluation

Client need: Physiological integrity

Clinical skill level: 2

■ After gastric surgery, the patient teaching includes:
1. Eat smaller meals
2. Avoid fluids with meals
3. Include complex carbohydrates
4. Avoid all saturated fats

Answer: 2. Avoid fluids with meals

Rationale: Fluid with food is believed to cause the "dumping syndrome" that often follows gastric surgery.

Nursing process: Intervention

Client need: Physiological integrity

Clinical skill level: 3

■ Which test does the nurse recognize as being specific for liver function?
1. ALT
2. HDL
3. LDH
4. Amylase

Answer: 1. ALT

Rationale: Of all the liver-associated aminotransferases, the ALT, (formerly SGPT) has relatively low concentrations in other tissues and hence is specific to the liver. Aminotransferase rises to levels that roughly parallel the extent of hepatocellular damage.

Nursing process: Assessment

Client need: Physiological integrity

Clinical skill level: 2

■ The physician orders enemas until clear. The nurse should restrict the total to three enemas because there is an electrolyte imbalance associated with excessive enemas. Which imbalance is of most concern?
1. Hypercalcemia
2. Hypocalcemia
3. Hyperkalemia
4. Hypokalemia

Answer: 4. Hypokalemia

Rationale: Repeated enemas cause imbalance of the potassium and sodium in the cell compartments, causing hypokalemia, hyponatremia and potential for water intoxication.

Nursing process: Evaluation

Client need: Physiological integrity

Clinical skill level: 2

■ What is the first-line treatment for a patient with pancreatitis?
1. Nasogastric suction
2. Enemas until clear
3. IV antibiotics
4. Morphine IV

Answer: 1. Nasogastric suction

Rationale: Management is directed toward inhibiting pancreatic activity, and suctioning decreases stimuli for release of gastric enzymes.

Nursing process: Intervention

Client need: Physiological integrity

Clinical skill level: 3

UNIT 10
MALE & FEMALE REPRODUCTIVE SYSTEMS

- Hysterectomy
- Ovarian Cancer
- Toxic Shock Syndrome
- Prostate Cancer
- Prostatitis
- Benign Prostatic Hyperplasia

HYSTERECTOMY

DEFINITION
A hysterectomy is a surgical procedure to remove female reproductive organs.

PATHOPHYSIOLOGY
Four types of hysterectomies may be performed:
- Subtotal hysterectomy
  - All of the uterus except the cervix is removed
- Total hysterectomy
  - Removal of the uterus and cervix either abdominally or vaginally
- Total abdominal hysterectomy with bilateral salpingo-oophorectomy
  - Removal of the uterus, cervix, fallopian tubes, ovaries
- Radical hysterectomy
  - Removal of the uterus, cervix, fallopian tubes, ovaries, lymph nodes, upper third of the vagina, parametrium

ASSOCIATED MEDICAL CONDITIONS
- Cancer
- Pulmonary embolus

ASSESSMENT
- Abnormal bleeding
- Minimal urinary output
- Decreased bowel sounds
- Bladder distention
- Depression
- Gas pains

NURSING INTERVENTIONS
- Strict I&O
- Catheterization as ordered
- Perineal Care
- Leg exercises to promote circulation
- Fluids orally
- Auscultate abdomen for flatus
- Rectal tube as ordered

PATIENT TEACHING
- Heavy lifting and physical exercise
- Loss of reproductive ability
- When sexual activity may be resumed

ASSOCIATED NURSING DIAGNOSES
- Activity intolerance, high risk for
- Anxiety
- Constipation
- Fear
- Infection, high risk for
- Powerlessness
- Urinary elimination, altered
- Family coping, compromised, ineffective
- Body image disturbance
- Fatigue
- Hopelessness
- Pain
- Role performance, altered

STUDY QUESTIONS

■ The patient is 7 hours post-hysterectomy. She has not been able to void since returning from surgery, and she does not have a Foley catherer. At what point will the nurse alert the physician?
1. 3-4 hours
2. 8-10 hours
3. 12-16 hours
4. 24 hours postop

Answer: 2. 8-10 hours

Rationale: If the patient has not voided in 8-10 hours with the assistance of traditional measures, then the physician should be notified. At that point, he will probably order insertion of a catheter.

Nursing process: Evaluation

Client need: Physiological integrity

Clinical skill level: 3

■ The hysterectomy patient who is 12 hours postop has been somewhat uncooperative in turning, coughing, and deep breathing and using the incentive spirometer. The nurse is concerned because the surgery was longer than expected, and the patient is obese. What is the first priority of care?
1. Postural drainage
2. Early ambulation
3. Slow IV fluids
4. Monitor temperature

Answer: 2. Early ambulation

Rationale: This patient is already at risk for complications, especially thrombus formation and pulmonary embolus. Ambulation and ROM is the key to prevention.

Nursing process: Intervention

Client need: Physiological integrity

Clinical skill level: 3

■ A 50-year-old obese woman is three days post-op following an abdominal hysterectomy. She is complaining of pain in her right calf. The nurse assesses a positive Homan's sign. Which nursing interventions should be avoided:
1. Putting on anti-embolic stocking
2. Elevation of the affected limb
3. Massaging the patient's legs
4. Active and passive ROM

Answer: 3. Massaging the patient's legs

Rationale: A positive Homan's sign is indicative of a thrombus. Massaging may cause it to break loose and become a dangerous embolism.

Nursing process: Intervention

Client need: Physiological integrity

Clinical skill level: 2

OVARIAN CANCER

DEFINITION
The leading cause of death from reproductive cancers, ovarian cancer is second only to uterine cancer in female gynecological malignancies. The disease has been linked to celibacy, nulliparity, infertility and endometriosis.

PATHOPHYSIOLOGY
The majority of ovarian cancers are epithelial tumors; others are adenocarcinomas. The cancer spreads asymptomatically until it leads to pressure on surrounding organs. By the time symptoms occur, the cancer has usually spread to the fallopian tubes, uterus, ligaments, and the other ovary, and may spread into the bowel omentum and other organs. The prognosis for ovarian cancer remains very poor in spite of new techniques for treatment.

ASSOCIATED MEDICAL CONDITIONS
- Terminal cancer

NURSING ASSESSMENT
- Indigestion (an early sign)
- Urinary frequency, urgency
- Pleural effusion
- Bowel dysfunction
- Abnormal uterine bleeding
- Abdominal distention (feeling of bloating)
- Abdominal pain (in later stages)
- Constipation
- Dyspnea
- Pain from pressure caused by tumor

CLIENT NEED
Physiological integrity

NURSING INTERVENTIONS
- Early detection:
  - Recognition of subtle signs and symptoms
  - Intravenous pyelogram

- Barium enema
- Ultrasound
- Provide psychological support
- Assist in total hysterectomy
- Refer to support groups, if possible
- Assist in chemotherapy, radiation therapy

PATIENT TEACHING

- New medications that are available for ovarian cancer
- Refer to hospice when appropriate
- Teach family and significant others how to be emotionally supportive
- Patients who have completed chemotherapy and are free of cancer should have follow-up laparotomy to determine whether further treatment is necessary

ASSOCIATED NURSING DIAGNOSES

- Anxiety
- Hopelessness
- Family coping, disabling, ineffective
- Pain
- Sexual patterns, altered
- Constipation
- Grieving, anticipatory
- Nutrition: less than body requirements, altered
- Powerlessness
- Spiritual distress

STUDY QUESTIONS

■ In taking a patient history, the nurse realizes that the woman at highest risk for ovarian cancer is the woman who:
1. Began regular periods at age 14
2. Was never able to have children
3. Experienced menopause at age 52
4. Has a life-long history of smoking

Answer: 2. Was never able to have children

Rationale: The highest incidence of ovarian cancer is among women who have never been pregnant, who began menstrual periods early (age 11, 12) and who experience early menopause.

Nursing process: Assessment

Client need: Physiological integrity

Clinical skill level: 2

■ A presenting symptom of ovarian cancer that could lead to early diagnosis is:
1. Indigestion, bloating
2. Urinary frequency, pain
3. Bleeding, abdominal pain
4. Pelvic discomfort, discharge

Answer: 1. Indigestion, bloating

Rationale: The vague symptoms of dyspepsia, inability to eat heavy meals, and bloating are early symptoms. Urinary frequency, constipation, and pelvic pressure present in later stages when ovarian cancer is usually diagnosed.

Nursing process: Assessment

Client need: Physiological integrity

Clinical skill level: 3

TOXIC SHOCK SYNDROME

DEFINITION
Toxic shock syndrome is caused by Staphylococcus aureaus. The poison can infect any part of the body and often affects several organ systems.

PATHOPHYSIOLOGY
TSS occurs in men, women and children but has been linked particular to super-absorbent tampon use because these tampons absorb large amounts of menstrual blood and may be left in place for longer period of time that other types of tampons. This creates a favorable environment in which the Staphylococcus aureaus can grow.

ASSOCIATED MEDICAL CONDITIONS
- Shock
- Disseminated intravascular coagulopathy (DIC)

ASSESSMENT
- High fever
- Diarrhea
- Hypotension
- Acidosis
- Vomiting
- Red, macular rash
- Monitor ABGs
- Shock lung

CLIENT NEED
- Physiological integrity

NURSING INTERVENTION
- Monitor strict I&O
- Observe for hematomas, cyanosis, petechiae
- Observe for bleeding at IV sites
- Monitor vital signs
- Monitor for compromised circulation

PATIENT TEACHING

- Use sanitary napkins at night, not tampons
- Change tampons regularly and insert carefully to prevent abrasions
- Utilize good handwashing techniques
- Female patients with a history of TSS should not use tampons until TSS bacteria is no longer present in vaginal flora

ASSOCIATED NURSING DIAGNOSES

- Anxiety
- Knowledge deficit
- Noncompliance
- Tissue perfusion, altered,
- Fear
- Health-seeking behavior
- Pain
- Body temperature, high risk for altered

STUDY QUESTIONS

■ The nurse is assessing a female patient, 16, for possible toxic shock syndrome. What is the first cardinal sign that signals this emergency?

1. Rapid onset of hypertension
2. Rapid onset of high fever
3. Sudden, sharp abdominal pain
4. Rapid onset of pelvic bleeding

Answer: 2. Rapid onset of high fever

Rationale: The toxicity of Staphyloccus aureus becomes obvious with the sudden high fever that is the initial sign of toxic shock syndrome. It most often occurs in women using highly-absorbent tampons.

Nursing process: Assessment

Client need: Physiological integrity

Clinical skill level: 2

■ The nurse is closely monitoring the patient with toxic shock syndrome, and is now assessing new signs of petechiae, cyanosis, and slight oozing of blood from the IV site. This alerts her to the complication of:
1. Septic shock
2. Shock lung
3. Vasogenic shock
4. Disseminated intravascular coagulopathy

Answer: 4. Disseminated intravascular coagulopathy

Rationale: DIC is a frequent complication of toxic shock. Other signs are development of hematomas and cold extremities.

Nursing process: Evaluation

Client need: Physiological integrity

Clinical skill level: 4

PROSTATITIS

DEFINITION
Prostatitis is an inflammation of the prostate gland which may be acute bacterial, chronic bacterial, or nonbacterial.

PATHOPHYSIOLOGY
Acute bacterial is the most common form of prostatitis. Acute bacterial prostatitis can occur following a viral illness or may occur along with a decrease in sexual activity. Bacterial prostatitis is associated with urinary tract infections.

ASSOCIATED MEDICAL CONDITIONS
- UTI
- Cystitis
- Epidiymitis
- Prostatic abscess
- Septicemia
- Pyelonephritis

ASSESSMENT
- Elevated WBC count
- Cloudy urine with foul odor

Acute prostatitis:
- High fever
- Dysuria
- Tender prostate
- Low back pain
- Chills
- Urethral discharge
- Nocturia
- Urinary retention

Chronic prostatitis
- Urinary dysfunction
- Muscle aches
- Backache

CLIENT NEED
Physiological integrity

NURSING INTERVENTIONS
- Administer antibiotic (tetracycline)
- Recommend sitz baths
- Administer pain medications
- Administer stool softners

- Prepare for intravenous pyelogram (IVP)
- Encourage bedrest
- Assess for allergies to iodine related to IVP

PATIENT TEACHING
- Maintain high fluid intake
- Report changes in I&O that may indicate urinary retention
- Take medication as prescribed

ASSOCIATED NURSING DIAGNOSES
- Anxiety
- Hopelessness
- Urinary retention
- Physical mobility, impaired
- Fear
- Pain
- Urinary elimination, altered

STUDY QUESTIONS

■ The patient with prostatitis asks why he has to avoid coffee, alcohol, and chocolate. The nurse tells him these foods have diuretic actions and cause:
1. Urinary retention
2. Urinary infection
3. Increased prostatic secretions
4. Increased prostatic spasms

Answer: 3. Increased prostatic secretions

Rationale: Foods that increase prostatic secretions and should be avoided also include tea, colas, and spices.

Nursing process: Intervention

Client need: Physiological integrity

Clinical skill level: 3

■ The nurse encourages regular fluid intake, but "forcing fluids" is not included in the plan of care for the patient with prostatitis. The rationale for this is to:
1. Maintain medication levels
2. Decrease urine output
3. Maintain balanced I&O
4. Prevent renal overload

Answer: 1. Maintain medication levels

Rationale: Forcing fluids might decrease levels of antimicrobials, such as tetracycline, doxycycline, or trimethoprime-sulfamethoxazole, that are often prescribed for prostatitis.

Nursing process: Intervention

Client need: Physiological integrity

Clinical skill level: 3

PROSTATE CANCER

DEFINITION
The third leading cause of death among men in the U.S., prostate cancer is the most common male cancer.

PATHOPHYSIOLOGY
Prostate tumors are usually androgen-dependent adenocarcinomas. The tumor originates in the posterior portions of the prostate and spreads to the seminal vesicles, urethral mucosa, external sphincter, perineural lymphatic system and lymph nodes.

ASSESSMENT
Early signs:
- Difficulty starting urination
- Urinary obstruction
- Hematuria
- Urinary retention
- Stool changes
- Pain radiating down hips and legs
- Cystitis without underlying cause
- Dribbling and retention
- Nocturia
- Hard, enlarged prostate
- Pain on defecation
- Elevated serum acid phosphate

CLIENT NEED
Physiological integrity

NURSING INTERVENTIONS
- Early detection of tumor
- Ultrasonography,
- Magnetic resonance imaging
- X-ray assessment
- CT scanning

After detection:
- Radiation therapy
- Endocrine therapy

- Administer estrogen (diethylstilbestrol) to reduce serum testosterone levels
- Assist in total prostatectomy

PATIENT TEACHING
- Kegel exercises to control incontinence
- Need for regular examinations

ASSOCIATED NURSING DIAGNOSES
- Anxiety
- Constipation
- Fear
- Urinary elimination, altered
- Pain, chronic
- Sexual dysfunction
- Hopelessness
- Body image disturbance
- Fatigue
- Grieving, anticipatory
- Nutrition: less than body requirements
- Powerlessness
- Urinary retention
- Spiritual distress, distress of the human spirit

STUDY QUESTIONS

■ In evaluating lab results, serum acid phosphate level is elevated in:
1. Chronic malnutrition
2. Chronic infection
3. Diabetic mellitus
4. Prostatic carcinoma

Answer: 4. Prostatic carcinoma

Rationale: The prostate contains roughly 1000 times more acid phosphate than does any other organ in the body. High serum acid phosphate levels are considered part of the diagnostic testing for metastatic prostate cancer.

Nursing process: Evaluation

Client need: Physiological integrity

| Clinical skill level: 3 |

■ A male, age 36, is diagnosed in the early stages of prostate cancer. He is considering the choice of treatments. The physician recommends radiation therapy, primarily because:
1. It is not invasive
2. There are few side effects
3. It is much more effective
4. The risk of impotency is decreased

Answer: 4. The risk of impotency is decreased
Rationale: With radiation therapy, the chance is much greater that sexual potency can be preserved than with surgery.
Nursing process: Intervention
Client need: Physiological integrity

Clinical skill level: 3

■ The patient returns to his room via recovery following a prostatectomy complaining of pain. Which action has priority?
1. Administering a narcotic
2. Checking catheter patency
3. Notifying the surgeon
4. Place in a modified Trendelenburg

Answer: 2. Checking catheter patency
Rationale: A common cause of pain following surgery is urinary retention caused by a blocked catheter.
Nursing process: Assessment
Client need: Physiological integrity

Clinical skill level: 3

BENIGN PROSTATIC HYPERPLASIA

DEFINITION
Benign prostatic hyperplasia the most common problem of the male reproductive system. The disorder occurs in approximately 50% of men over the age of 50 and 75% of men over the age of 70.

PATHOPHYSIOLOGY
As the patient ages, hyperplasia occurs in which an abnormal increase in the number of normal cells in the prostate takes place. As these cells grow, they compress the surrounding prostatic tissue and form an overgrowth of smooth muscle and connective tissue. Possible causes of the condition include excessive accumulation of dihydroxytestosterone in the prostate, estrogen stimulation, and local growth hormone. The enlarged prostate gland causes urinary obstruction which can lead to renal insufficiency.

ASSOCIATED MEDICAL CONDITIONS
- Urinary tract infections
- Renal failure

NURSING ASSESSMENT
- Urinary dysfunction
- Hematuria

NURSING INTERVENTIONS
- Assist in prostatectomy as ordered
- X-ray
- Catheterization to assess amount of residual urine

PATIENT TEACHING
- Patient should void as urge is felt
- Avoid alcohol because of diuretic effects
- Avoid consuming large quantities of liquid
- Avoid medications containing phenylpropanolamine and phenylephrine as these will worsen the condition

ASSOCIATED NURSING DIAGNOSES
- Anxiety
- Fatigue
- Incontinence, urge
- Pain
- Sexual patterns, altered
- Urinary retention
- Constipation
- Hopelessness
- Incontinence, total
- Powerlessness
- Social isolation

STUDY QUESTIONS

■ A 65 year-old man with a history of hypertension and prostatic hyperplasia is admitted with an acute urinary retention and is scheduled for a transurethral prostatectomy (TURP). Nursing care focuses on:
1. Decreasing hypertension
2. Encouraging fluid intake
3. Providing gradual drainage of urine
4. Administering anticoagulant therapy

Answer: 3. Providing gradual drainage of urine

Rationale: The patient with benign prostatic hyperplasia is usually admitted because he is unable to void due to obstruction. Catheterization is a priority.

Nursing process: Intervention

Client need: Physiological integrity

Clinical skill level: 2

- The nurse instructs the patient that a transurethral resection of the prostate involves:
  1. A low abdominal incision
  2. An incision into the anus
  3. Placement of a suprapubic catheter
  4. Use of an endoscopic device into the penis

  Answer: 4. Use of an endoscopic device into the penis
  Rationale: This instrument is used to view the prostate as well as remove the gland with an electrical cutting loop.
  Nursing process: Intervention
  Client need: Physiological integrity

  Clinical skill level: 3

UNIT 11
THE EYE & EAR

- Cataracts
- Glaucoma
- Meniere's Disease
- Otitis Media

CATARACTS

DEFINITION
The opaqueness covering the lens of the eye, usually caused by the aging process, chronic infection, or diabetes mellitus.

PATHOPHYSIOLOGY
Although new fiber cells replenish the lens throughout the individual's lifetime, by the age of seventy this process has slowed significantly. The lens becomes opaque as the result of the deterioration of its molecules from a lifetime of ultraviolet radiation. Abnormal fluorescent substances form in the aging lens which result in yellowing.

ASSESSMENT
- Gradual loss of sight
- Blurred vision
- Opaqueness of lens

CLIENT NEED
Physiological integrity

INTERVENTION
- Provide safety related to loss of vision
- Administer antibiotics and/or analgesics
- Tell patient not to touch eyes or patch
- Prevent increase in intraocular pressure, especially postoperatively

MEDICAL INTERVENTIONS
- Surgery, usually laser
- Prescribe mydriatics before surgery

PATIENT TEACHING
- Avoid quick movements
- Notify physician of sudden onset of pain
- No bending or stooping
- May indicate hemorrhage or suture rupture

ASSOCIATED NURSING DIAGNOSES
- Anxiety
- Injury, high risk for
- Home maintenance management, impaired
- Body image disturbance
- Hopelessness
- Self-care deficit: bathing/hygiene, dressing/grooming, feeding, toileting

STUDY QUESTIONS

■ The nurse tells the patient that she will be putting two drops of medication in his eyes. She instructs, "After I put the drops in your eyes, please . . ."
1. Gently close your eyes"
2. Squeeze your eyes shut"
3. Keep your eyes open"
4. Put this cloth over your eyes"

Answer: 1. Gently close your eyes"

Rationale: If the eyes are not closed gently, the medication will be expelled. Keeping the eyes closed will prevent the eye from removing the liquid through a natural reflex action.

Nursing process: Intervention

Client need: Physiological integrity

Clinical skill level: 2

■ Eye medications that dilate the pupils are:
1. Miotics
2. Mydriatics
3. Osmotics
4. Inhibitors

Answer: 2. Mydriatics

Rationale: One of the reasons the mydriatics are prescribed is because the physician wants the eyes to be dilated. Mydriatics paralyze the ciliary muscle of the iris causing pupillary dilation.

Nursing process: Outcome criteria

Client need: Physiological integrity

Clinical skill level: 2

■ A physician who performs eye surgery may prescribe a topical mydriatic postoperatively because it:
1. Constricts the pupil
2. Dilates the pupil
3. Decreases dizziness
4. Fights infection

Answer: 2. Dilates the pupil

Rationale: The mydriatic, such as atropine, facilitates examination of the eye, particularly the retina and the optic disc. It also decreases irritation if the eye is infected.

Nursing process: Outcome criteria

Client need: Physiological integrity

Clinical skill level: 2

■ Two different eye medications are to be administered. These medications must be instilled:
1. At the same time
2. About 5 minutes apart
3. About 30 minutes apart
4. About 1 hour apart

Answer: 2. About 5 minutes apart

Rationale: The eye can hold only one drop at a time. A period of about 5 minutes between medications will allow the eye to adequately absorb the first medication and prevent any potential interactions between the two medications.

Nursing process: Intervention

Client need: Physiological integrity

Clinical skill level: 2

■ In assessing the eye the examiner inspects the lens. The lens is normally:
1. Shiny
2. Thick
3. Opaque
4. Transparent

Answer: 4. Transparent

Rationale: The nurse should suspect an abnormal condition if the lens is not transparent.

Nursing process: Assessment

Client need: Health promotion and maintenance

Clinical skill level: 1

- When the lens is opaque, the patient has:
    1. Normal vision
    2. Cataracts
    3. Glaucoma
    4. Astigmatism

    Answer: 2. Cataracts

    Rationale: The opaque lens instead of the normal transparent lens is the cardinal sign of cataracts.

    Nursing process: Assessment

    Client need: Health promotion and maintenance

    Clinical skill level: 1

- Visual acuity means:
    1. Ability to pass a driving test
    2. Accuracy of vision
    3. Irregularities in visual fields
    4. Ability to read

    Answer: 2. Accuracy of vision

    Rationale: Acuity means how well the person can see.

    Nursing process: Assessment

    Client need: Health promotion and maintenance

    Clinical skill level: 1

GLAUCOMA

DEFINITION
Increased intraocular pressure caused by a decreased outflow of aqueous humor into the canal of Schlemm.

PATHOPHYSIOLOGY
The optic nerve atrophies as a result of increase in intraocular pressure which damages the nerve fibers in the retina.

ASSESSMENT
- Hardening eyeball
- Halos around lights
- Blind spots, especially in peripheral vision
- Dilated pupils
- Nausea and vomiting
- Blurred vision, progressive over a period of time

CLIENT NEED
Physiological integrity

NURSING INTERVENTIONS
Safety precautions

MEDICAL INTERVENTIONS
- Surgery may be required
- Prescribe miotic drugs to facilitate drainage of aqueous humor

PATIENT TEACHING
- Importance of regular exams
- Avoid situations that increase intraocular pressure such as stress, tight clothes around
- Continue to take prescribed medication

neck, lifting and respiratory infection

NURSING DIAGNOSES
- Activity intolerance,
- Home maintenance management, impaired
- Fear
- Physical mobility, impaired
- Self-Care Deficit: bathing/hygiene, dressing/grooming, feeding, toileting
- Anxiety
- Coping, ineffective individual
- Knowledge deficit
- Sensory/perceptual alterations: olfactory

STUDY QUESTIONS

■ A patient who is partially blind has been diagnosed with open-angle glaucoma. The goal of treatment in glaucoma is:
1. Decrease aqueous humor
2. Increase aqueous humor
3. Decrease discomfort
4. Restore vision

Answer: 1. Decrease aqueous humor

Rationale: The goal of treatment is to decrease aqueous humor, thus decreasing intraocular pressure, and to slow the condition enough to maintain good eye vision.

Nursing process: Outcome criteria

Client need: Physiological integrity

Clinical skill level: 2

- The patient has been complaining of headache and dull, persistent pain in the eye. Another cardinal symptom common to glaucoma is:
    1. Lacrimation
    2. Fixed pupil
    3. Reddened cornea
    4. Halos around lights

    Answer: 4. Halos around lights

    Rationale: A rapid rise in corneal edema causes halo vision, in which the patient sees colored halos around lights. Other signs are blurred vision and redness.

    Nursing process: Assessment

    Client need: Physiological integrity

    Clinical skill level: 2

- The patient asks the nurse, "What is glaucoma?" The nurse bases her answer on the pathophysiologic basis of glaucoma, which is:
    1. Clouding of lens
    2. Infection of cornea
    3. Separation of the retinal layers
    4. Obstruction of aqueous humor drainage

    Answer: 4. Obstruction of aqueous humor drainage

    Rationale: Glaucoma is damage that is caused by an excess of aqueous humor, or obstruction to aqueous outflow that leads to increased optical pressure (IOP). The higher the pressure, the more damage to the eye.

    Nursing process: Intervention

    Client need: Physiological integrity

    Clinical skill level: 2

- Eye medications that contract the pupil are:
  1. Mydriatics
  2. Miotics
  3. Osmotics
  4. Inhibitors

  Answer: 2. Miotics

  Rationale: Mydriatics facilitate the examination of the optic disc and retina by putting the ciliary body at rest. Miotics cause constriction of the pupils through contraction of the ciliary muscle.

  Nursing process: Outcome criteria

  Client need: Physiological integrity

  Clinical skill level: 2

- The patient with glaucoma is prescribed a miotic medication, Pilocarpine. Patient teaching emphasizes that this medication:
  1. Is potentially addictive
  2. Causes digestion problems
  3. Has many drug interactions
  4. Must be taken for life

  Answer: 4. Must be taken for life

  Rationale: Since there is no cure for glaucoma, therefore, the medication cannot be discontinued.

  Nursing process: Outcome criteria

  Client need: Physiological integrity

  Clinical skill level: 2

- The patient taking Pilocarpine is instructed to instill drops just before going to bed because it causes:
    1. Disorientation
    2. Dizziness
    3. Drowsiness
    4. Blurred vision

    Answer: 3. Blurred vision

    Rationale: One of the major side-effects of Pilocarpine is blurred vision. It may also cause eye pain or irritation. If necessary, the antidote is atropine.

    Nursing process: Outcome criteria

    Client need: Physiological integrity

    Level of clinical skill: 3

- The action of Pilocarpine on the pupil is:
    1. Dilation
    2. Contraction
    3. Difficult to detect
    4. Not significant

    Answer: 2. Contraction

    Rationale: This medication increases aqueous humor into the outflow channels and reduces intraocular pressure through contraction of the pupil. The result is a decreased IOP.

    Nursing process: Outcome criteria

    Client need: Physiological integrity

    Clinical skill level: 2

MÉNIÈRE'S SYNDROME

DEFINITION
A dysfunction of the labyrinth that causes loss of equilibrium.

PATHOPHYSIOLOGY
The cause is unknown, but may be related to infections, emotional stress, or genetic factors, allergies

ASSOCIATED MEDICAL CONDITIONS
- Vertigo

ASSESSMENT
- Dizziness/vertigo
- Headache
- Attacks are abrupt, but intermittent
- Nausea and vomiting (related to vertigo)
- Tinnitus
- Hearing loss
- Feeling of fullness caused by edema or inner ear

CLIENT NEED
Physiological integrity

NURSING INTERVENTIONS
- Bedrest during acute attacks
- Administer diuretics
- Instruct patient to move slowly as fast movements could initiate an attack
- Administer lidocaine
- Administer anticholinergics
- Recommend low-sodium diet
- Provide for safety
- Administer tranquilizers
- Surgery may be offered where medical therapy is ineffective

PATIENT TEACHING

- Avoid electrolyte imbalances, patient should distribute food intake throughout the day
- Avoid high solute foods containing salt and simple sugars which cause osmotic shifts.

ASSOCIATED NURSING DIAGNOSES

- Hopelessness
- Injury, high risk for
- Activity intolerance, high risk for
- Anxiety
- Social interaction, impaired

STUDY QUESTIONS

■ The patient diagnosed with Meniere's disease is prescribed diuretics. The rationale for this is:
  1. To decrease total body fluid
  2. To decrease total body weight
  3. To increase total output
  4. To decrease fluid in the inner ear

Answer: 4. To decrease fluid in the inner ear

Rationale: The patient with Meniere's will complain of fullness and ringing in the ear (tinnitus). A diuretic may relieve this condition.

Nursing process: Intervention

Client need: Physiological integrity

> Clinical skill level: 3

■ The priority nursing responsibility for a patient who is dizzy is:
1. Safety
2. Comfort
3. Hygiene
4. Nausea

Answer: 1. Safety

Rationale: The dizzy patient is constantly in danger of falling.

Nursing process: Intervention

Client need: Physiological integrity

Clinical skill level: 2

■ The nurse teaches the patient with vertigo to:
1. Avoid sudden movements
2. Avoid loud noises
3. Avoid walking or standing
4. Lie on affected side

Answer: 1. Avoid sudden movements

Rationale: Sudden movements will aggravate the dizziness by quickly throwing the body's equilibrium out of balance.

Nursing process: Intervention

Client need: Health promotion and maintenance

Clinical skill level: 2

- The cardinal symptom of Méniere's disease is:
    1. Earache
    2. Infection
    3. Vertigo
    4. Headaches

    Answer: 3. Vertigo

    Rationale: The diagnosis of Méniere's disease is based on a triad of symptoms which are whirling vertigo that causes nausea and vomiting, tinnitus, and loss of hearing. The vertigo is the first, and usually the most debilitating, symptom.

    Nursing process: Assessment

    Client need: Physiological integrity

    Clinical skill level: 2

OTITIS MEDIA

DEFINITION
An inflammation of the middle ear, common in childhood.

PATHOPHYSIOLOGY
An organism enters the auditory canal through the eustachian tube or through a perforated eardrum.

ASSOCIATED MEDICAL CONDITIONS
- Vertigo
- Pain

ASSESSMENT
- Severe earache
- Fever
- Headache
- Poor appetite
- Soreness over mastoid area
- Tinnitus
- Vertigo
- Nausea and vomiting

CLIENT NEED
Physiological integrity

NURSING INTERVENTIONS
- Administer pain medications
- Decrease fever
- Administer antibiotics
- Control nausea and vomiting

PATIENT TEACHING
- Instruct family on early signs of infection
- Give antibiotics for full course prescribed

ASSOCIATED NURSING DIAGNOSES
- Fatigue
- Body temperature, high risk for altered
- Sleep pattern disturbance
- Pain
- Sensory/perceptual alterations: auditory

General Study Questions

■ The priority nursing intervention when a foreign object is lodged in the cornea is:
1. Remove the object swiftly
2. Cover loosely with patch and consult physician
3. Wrap index finger with sterile gauze and wipe out
4. Irrigate with 1000 cc normal saline to remove object

Answer: 2. Cover loosely with patch and consult physician

Rationale: The cornea can be easily injured, and if not treated properly, moderate to severe vision loss could occur. A foreign object should never be removed by anyone but a doctor.

Nursing process: Intervention

Client need: Physiological integrity

Clinical skill level: 2

■ A welder suffers a burn to his eyes while welding late one afternoon. This kind of burn is:
1. A chemical burn
2. An ultraviolet burn
3. A thermal burn
4. A sun burn

Answer: 2. An ultraviolet burn

Rationale: The pain of this burn is not experienced upon contact, and the welder may not even realize he has sustained a burn until several hours later.

Nursing process: Assessment

Client need: Physiological integrity

Clinical skill level: 2

- The priority nursing intervention for the patient suffering a burn while welding is treatment of:
  1. Infection
  2. Abrasions
  3. Corneal ulcer
  4. Intense pain

  Answer: 4. Intense pain

  Rationale: The pain of a welding burn is so excruciating that medication must be instilled into the eye before assessment and other interventions can be conducted.

  Nursing process: Intervention

  Client need: Physiological integrity

  Clinical skill level: 2

- In assessing injury to the cornea, a dye is applied to the eye and then rinsed with saline. How is the site of injury detected?
  1. The dye is rinsed away completely
  2. The injured eye tissue remains stained
  3. The dye turns blue on the injured tissue
  4. The dye turns red on the injured tissue

  Answer: 2. The injured eye tissue remains stained

  Rationale: The dye that is placed in the eye will remain only on the part of the eye that is injured. Fluorescein sodium has an affinity for epithelium and vitreous of the eye. When exposed to UV light, injured tissues are seen as green or red.

  Nursing process: Assessment

  Client need: Physiological integrity

  Clinical skill level: 3

■ The initial priority of nursing interventions immediately following a chemical burn of the eye is:
1. Transport to a physician
2. Cover eyes with a cloth
3. Irrigate copiously with normal saline
4. Irrigate with anesthetic solution

Answer: 3. Irrigate copiously with normal saline

Rationale: The saline removes the chemical from the eyes, thereby relieving some of the pain and decreasing the possibility of further damage.

Nursing process: Intervention

Client need: Physiological integrity

| Clinical skill level: 2 |

■ What type of hearing loss results from otosclerosis?
1. Conductive
2. Fluctuant
3. Sensorineural
4. Sudden

Answer: 1. Conductive

Rationale: Otosclerosis is caused by the growth of abnormal spongy bone in the labyrinth. It eventually damages the stapes, and therefore, sound cannot vibrate through the ear.

Nursing process: Assessment

Client need: Physiological integrity

| Clinical skill level: 1 |

- How will the nurse facilitate communication with the hearing impaired?
    1. By smiling frequently
    2. By speaking loudly
    3. By talking directly into "best" ear
    4. By not overaccentuating words

    Answer: 4. By not overaccentuating words

    Rationale: The patient who has impaired hearing understands best when words are carefully annunciated at a normal tone of voice.

    Nursing process: Assessment

    Client need: Health promotion and maintenance

    Clinical skill level: 2

- Eye medications administered to a patient with corneal ulcers are:
    1. Miotics
    2. Mydriatics
    3. Non-steroid narcotics
    4. Corticosteroids

    Answer: 2. Mydriatics

    Rationale: Atropine or scopolamine are used to dilate the pupil, which in turn, prevents adhesions of the iris with the cornea.

    Nursing process: Intervention

    Client need: Physiological integrity

    Clinical skill level: 3

■ Post-surgery, which treatment is generally required for the patient suffering from a detached retina?
1. Bandage on operative eye
2. Bandage on both eyes
3. Cover good eye with shield
4. Neither eye should be bandaged

Answer: 2. Bandage on both eyes

Rationale: By bandaging both eyes, the tendency to blink and irritate either eye is decreased.

Nursing process: Intervention

Client need: Physiological integrity

Clinical skill level: 3

■ The nurse is using a vibrating tuning fork shifted between the mastoid bone and an area 2 inches from the canal opening of the ear. Which test is she performing?
1. Weber test
2. Rinne test
3. Schwabach test
4. Taylor test

Answer: 2. Rinne test

Rationale: This test is done to compare conductive hearing with sensorineural.

Nursing process: Outcome criteria

Client need: Physiological integrity

Clinical skill level: 2

■ The patient is complaining of dizziness. The nurse considers the ear structure that maintains a sense of equilibrium, which is:
1. External ear
2. Middle ear
3. Inner ear
4. Tympanic membrane

Answer: 3. Inner ear

Rationale: The labyrinth contains the organs of balance which are located in the inner ear.

Nursing process: Evaluation

Client need: Physiological integrity

Clinical skill level: 2

■ An important nursing intervention when testing distance vision with the Snellen Chart is to instruct the patient to:
1. Use both eyes to read the chart
2. Read the chart from right to left
3. Cover one eye while testing the other
4. Test only one eye since they will be the same

Answer: 3. Cover one eye while testing the other

Rationale: The Snellen test will evaluate the distance that each eye can recognize a letter or symbol.

Nursing process: Assessment

Client need: Health promotion and maintenance

Clinical skill level: 2

- Decreased flexibility of the lens is common as a person ages. This decreased ability to accommodate for detailed work is called:
    1. Senility
    2. Refraction
    3. Presbyopia
    4. Myopia

    Answer: 3. Presbyopia

    Rationale: The person usually notes presbyopia in the late 40s and begin to use "reading glasses."

    Nursing process: Assessment

    Client need: Health promotion and maintenance

    Clinical skill level: 1

- When the eye adjusts to seeing objects at various distances, it is called:
    1. PERLA
    2. Refraction
    3. Focusing
    4. Accommodation

    Answer: 4. Accommodation

    Rationale: Accommodation is tested by moving the index finger from side to side, back and forth, up and down to assess if the eyes follow the path of movement.

    Nursing process: Assessment

    Client need: Health promotion and maintenance

    Clinical skill level: 1

■ In assessing a patient, the nurse realizes the cardinal symptom of an inner ear problem is:
1. Echoing voices
2. Headache pain
3. Dizziness
4. Hearing loss

Answer: 3. Dizziness

Rationale: The inner ear controls the equilibrium of the body, and if there is a problem of the inner ear the patient will experience dizziness.

Nursing process: Assessment

Client need: Physiological integrity

Clinical skill level: 2

■ Upon visualization with an otoscope, the healthy tympanic membrane is:
1. Pinkish, translucent
2. Pearly gray, translucent
3. Shiny white, glowing
4. Increasing respirations, pulse rate

Answer: 2. Pearly gray, translucent

Rationale: If the membrane is shiny, glowing, or bulging, the patient may have an ear infection.

Nursing process: Assessment

Client need: Physiological integrity

Clinical skill level: 1

UNIT 12
CONCEPTS OF SPECIAL CONCERN

- Burns
- Cancer
- Hemorrhage
- Hypovolemic Shock
- Informed Consent
- Lead Poisoning
- Malignant Hyperthermia
- Pain
- Shock

BURNS

DEFINITION
A burn is an injury which results from direct exposure to a thermal, chemical, electrical or radiation source resulting in the transfer of the energy to body tissues. The degree of heat and length of time exposed determines the degree of injury.

PATHOPHYSIOLOGY
In cases of minor burns, only the local area responds to the injury. For burns exceeding 25% of the total body surface area, the body responds proportionately to the extent of the injury. In cases involving major burn injuries, all major body systems respond.

Burns are classified according to risk of death and disfiguration or disability. The following factors determine burn severity:
- Burn depth, according to degree or depth of skin burned:
  - Superficial partial thickness (First degree): Epidermis is blistered. Example: Sunburn
  - Deep partial thickness (Second degree): Epidermis and dermis are damaged. Wound is very red, quite painful and exudates fluid. Example: Scalding with hot water.
  - Full-thickness (Third degree): Epidermis, dermis, and underlying tissues are destroyed. Wound is painless because all nerve tissue has been destroyed, and may vary from white to black.
- Burn size
- Burn location
- Client age

ASSOCIATED MEDICAL CONDITIONS
- Hypovolemic Shock
- Smoke Inhalation
- Septic Shock
- Carbon Monoxide Poisoning

ASSESSMENT
- Blister formation
- Chills resulting from heat loss, anxiety, pain
- Minimal urine output
- Thirst
- Severe pain in superficial partial thickness burns
- Anesthesia in full and deep partial thickness burns

- Inhalation injury
  - Facial and neck burns
  - Swelling of nasopharynx
  - Wheezing
  - Sooty sputum

CLIENT NEED
Physiological integrity

NURSING INTERVENTIONS
- Assess vital signs
- Eliminate source of burn if possible
- Note baseline laboratory studies
- Assess for soot in sputum
- Start IV where possible
- Administer fluid replacement
- Administer narcotic analgesics IV
- Assess for hypothermia
- Administer pain relief
- Ensure airway, sufficient breathing, circulation
- Remove dead tissue, clean debris from wound
- Assess depth, severity of burn
- Administer tetanus toxoid
- Immerse in cold water (minor burns only)
- Apply topical medications, when ordered

PATIENT TEACHING
- Need for physical therapy during rehabilitation phase
- Understanding of limitations posed by burns
- Use of lotions and creams with dressing to protect and moisten wound

ASSOCIATED NURSING DIAGNOSES

- Coping, defensive
- Airway clearance, ineffective
- Fear
- Hopelessness
- Gas exchange, impaired
- Tissue perfusion, cerebral, cardiopulmonary, peripheral
- Pain
- Post-trauma response
- Nutrition, less than body requirements, altered
- Body image disturbance
- Coping, ineffective individual
- Fluid volume deficit
- Hyperthermia
- Infection, high risk for
- Self-care deficit, bathing/hygiene, dressing/grooming, feeding, toileting
- Physical mobility, impaired
- Skin integrity, impaired
- Management of therapeutic regime, individual, ineffective

STUDY QUESTIONS

■ Electrical burns can cause multiple injuries. The injury most likely to cause death is:
1. Depression of respirations
2. Internal tissue damage
3. Multiple bone fractures
4. Ventricular fibrillation

Answer: 4. Ventricular fibrillation

Rationale: The electrical shock causes the myocardial tissue to "quiver" instead of contract. Cardiac output ceases. CPR is required.

Nursing process: Assessment

Client need: Physiological integrity

| Clinical skill level: 3 |

■ Edema is a common complication in burns. What is the cause of this edema?
1. Generalized capillary fluid pressure
2. Shift in capillary oncotic pressure
3. Increase in capillary oncotic pressure
4. Decrease in capillary oncotic pressure

Answer: 2. Shift in capillary oncotic pressure

Rationale: The cells that are destroyed release substances that increase capillary permeability, leading to massive fluid loss from the intravascular space into the interstitial spaces. Edema occurs in this interstitial space.

Nursing process: Evaluation

Client need: Physiological integrity

Clinical skill level: 3

■ Staphylococcus aureus has been cultured from the wound of a burn patient. The nurse implements which category of isolation?
1. Strict
2. Reverse
3. Enteric
4. Respiratory

Answer: 1. Strict

Rationale: Staphylococcus aureus is a highly communicable pathogen, and strict isolation is required to protect the patient.

Nursing process: Intervention

Client need: Physiological integrity

Level of clinical skill: 2

CANCER

DEFINITION

The word "cancer" is an umbrella word for many different diseases that begin at the cellular level and often proliferate to tissues and organs.

PATHOPHYSIOLOGY

Carcinogenesis is characterized by the development of abnormal cell structure and proliferate growth of abnormal cells. There are several theories of what causes this cell growth, ranging from specific carcinogens and viruses that cause cancer to environmental and immunologic factors. Malignant tumors are categorized according to a system of grading, classification, and staging. This information describes the extent of the malignancy and is often the basis of treatment.

Grading ranges from I to IV, with Grade I having the best prognosis and Grade IV having the poorest. Prognosis grading is done on the basis of differentiation, or how closely the cancer cell resembles the normal cell. A well-differentiated cell (Grade I) resembles the normal cell and the poorly-differentiated cell (Grade IV) is anaplastic. Classification of a tumor refers to the tissue where the malignancy originates. Basically there are two classifications: Carcinomas (skin, mucous membranes, glands) and sarcomas (bone, blood, lymphatics, connective tissue).

The TNM system is used. T stands for tumor, N for nodes, and M for metastasis:

- T:
  - The characteristics of the primary tumor, including size and involvement of surrounding tissue. On a scale of T0 to T4.
- N:
  - Spread to lymph nodes. On a scale of N0 to N3.
- M:
- Degree of metastasis.
  - On a scale of M0 (no metastasis) to M1 (metastatic involvement).

ASSOCIATED MEDICAL CONDITIONS
- Lung cancer
- Colon cancer
- Malignant melanoma
- Prostate cancer
- Breast cancer
- Ovarian cancer
- Leukemia
- Lymphoma

ASSESSMENT
- Change in appetite
- Sore that will not heal
- Night sweats
- Nausea and vomiting
- Diarrhea
- Stomatitis
- Fatigue
- Fever
- Pain
- Constipation
- Anemia

CLIENT NEED
Physiological integrity

MEDICAL INTERVENTIONS
Prescribe chemotherapy:
- **Antimetabolites:**
  - Cytosine arabinoside (Cytosar)
  - Methotrexate (Mexate)
  - 5 Fluorouracil (5 FU)
  - 6-Mercaptopurine (6-MP)
  - 6-Thioguanine (6-TG)

Alkylating agents:
- Busulfan (Mylcran)
- Chlorambucil (Leukeran)
- Dacarbazine (DTIC)
- Melphalan (Alkeran, L-PAM)
- Thiotepa
- Carmustine (BCNU)
- Cyclophosphamide (Cytoxan)
- Lomustine (CCNU)
- Nitrogen mustard (Mustargen)

Plant alkaloids:
- Etoposide (VePesid;VP-16)
- Vincristine (Oncovin)
- Vinblastine (Velban)

Antibiotics
- Bleomycin (Blenoxane)
- Doxorubicin (Adriamycin)
- Streptozocin (Streptozotocin)
- Mitomycin C (Mutamycin)
- Daunorubicin (Cerubidine)
- Mithramycin (Mithracin)
- Actinomycin D (Dactinomycin, Cosmegen)

PATIENT TEACHING
- Teach dangers of cigarette smoking
- Teach dangers of drinking alcohol
- **Teach anti-cancer dietary habits:**
  - Reduce total fats, both saturated and unsaturated
  - Eat fruits, especially citrus
  - Eat vegetables, especially cruciferons and those high in beta-carotene
  - Minimize intake of salt-cured or smoked foods
- Teach self-exams, as appropriate
- Encourage regular check-ups, depending upon age
- **Teach the warning signs of cancer:**
  - Change in bowel or bladder
  - Sore that does not heal
  - Unusual bleeding or discharge
  - Thickening or lump in the breast or elsewhere
  - Indigestion or difficulty in swallowing
  - Obvious change in wart or mole
  - Nagging cough or hoarseness

ASSOCIATED NURSING DIAGNOSES
- Anxiety
- Constipation
- Social isolation
- Body image disturbance
- Coping, ineffective individual
- Fatigue

- Fear
- Hopelessness
- Knowledge deficit
- Nutrition: less than body requirements, altered
- Powerlessness
- Family coping, compromised, ineffective
- Skin integrity, impaired
- Grieving, anticipatory
- Infection, high risk for
- Pain
- Management of therapeutic regime (individual), ineffective
- Role performance, altered
- Spiritual distress (distress of the human spirit)

STUDY QUESTIONS

■ In planning the care of a cancer patient with stomatitis, the nurse recommends:
1. A 1:1 solution of peroxide and water
2. A commercial mouthwash
3. A solution of mouthwash and peroxide
4. A solution of mouthwash and water

Answer: 1. A 1:1 solution of peroxide and water

Rationale: The peroxide solution will be less irritating. The over-the-counter mouthwashes may contain sodium or alcohol.

Nursing process: Intervention

Client need: Physiological integrity

Clinical skill level: 2

- The physician stages cancer as T4, N3, M1. The nurse recognizes this as:
  1. No metastasis
  2. Small tumor, no lymph involvement, no metastasis
  3. Large tumor, some lymph involvement, minimal metastasis
  4. Large tumor, advanced lymph enlargement with metastasis

  Answer: 4. Large tumor, advanced lymph enlargement with metastasis

  Rationale: T indicates size of tumor and its involvement with surrounding tissue, with T4 most advanced. N3 is indicative of advanced node involvement. M1 indicates metastasis.

  Nursing process: Evaluation

  Client need: Physiological integrity

  Clinical skill level: 3

- Which food would be recommended for a cancer patient who is on a high-protein, high-calorie diet?
  1. Skim-milk drinks
  2. Iced tea, fruit punch
  3. Red meat, vegetables
  4. Custard and jello

  Answer: 4. Custard and jello

  Rationale: Custard (with milk and eggs) is high in protein and calories. Jello is high in protein.

  Nursing process: Intervention

  Client need: Physiological integrity

  Clinical skill level: 3

- The nurse assesses white patches in the mouth of a cancer patient on chemotherapy. This is most likely:
  1. Candida infection
  2. Radiation damage
  3. Side-effect of antifungal medication
  4. Complication of eating citrus fruits

  Answer: 1. Candida infection

  Rationale: White patches adhering to the mucous membranes of the mouth is the cardinal sign of candida, which is a common side effect of chemotherapy.

  Nursing process: Assessment

  Client need: Physiological integrity

  Clinical skill level: 2

- The most common skin cancer generally appears on sun-exposed areas of the body. It is:
  1. Malignant melanoma
  2. Basal cell carcinoma
  3. Squamous cell carcinoma
  4. In situ cell carcinoma

  Answer: 2. Basal cell carcinoma

  Rationale: This carcinoma is the result of chronic exposure to UV light that leads to a mutant proliferation of basal (generative) cells of the skin. It can be cured if detected early.

  Nursing process: Assessment

  Client need: Physiological integrity

  Clinical skill level: 3

■ The cancer patient is prescribed an alkylating agent. The nurse teaches that alkylating agents are chemotherapy drugs that act by:
1. Preventing DNA replication
2. Preventing RNA replication
3. Interfering with cell synthesis
4. Interfering with cell transcription

Answer: 1. Preventing DNA replication
Rationale: Cancer chemotherapy is classified according to the way the drug acts on the cells.
Nursing process: Intervention
Client need: Physiological integrity

Clinical skill level: 3

■ The patient who is suffering alopecia as a side effect of chemotherapy is instructed that:
1. The hair loss is permanent
2. The hair will grow back after treatment
3. Drugs will be necessary to stimulate hair growth
4. There is no known remedy for hair loss

Answer: 2. The hair will grow back after treatment
Rationale: It usually takes about six weeks for hairs to grow back.
Nursing process: Intervention
Client need: Physiological integrity

Clinical skill level: 2

- The cancer patient is prescribed a course of chemotherapy. Patient teaching includes the information that radiation therapy works on the premise that:
  1. Malignant cells are more sensitive to radiation
  2. X-rays are strong enough to eliminate malignant cells
  3. Therapeutic doses kill only cancer and not normal cells
  4. X-rays are selective enough to destroy only malignant cells

  Answer: 1. Malignant cells are more sensitive to radiation

  Rationale: Radiation therapy kills both malignant cells and normal cells. However, malignant cells multiply at a much faster rate than normal cells, making them more susceptible to destruction.

  Nursing process: Evaluation

  Client need: Physiological integrity

  Clinical skill level: 3

- For the patient undergoing a course of external radiation treatments, the nurse should be alert for:
  1. Impairment of skin integrity
  2. Decreased mobility
  3. Constipation
  4. Ulceration of mucous membranes

  Answer: 1. Impairment of skin integrity

  Rationale: Radiation injures tissues and vessels supplying blood to tissues. Specific problems include erythema, peeling of the epidermis, and atrophy.

  Nursing process: Assessment

  Client need: Physiological integrity

  Clinical skill level: 2

■ A patient, 53, diagnosed with breast cancer is admitted to the hospital experiencing severe pain. The physician has ordered 2 to 10 mg morphine PO or IM prn for pain. Initially, the nurse will administer:
1. 2 mg IM
2. 2 mg PO
3. 5 mg IM
4. 10 mg IM

Answer: 4. 10 mg IM

Rationale: When pain is severe, initially the largest dosage should be administered when pain begins to abate, then dosages can be tapered.

Nursing process: Intervention

Client need: Physiological integrity

Clinical skill level: 3

■ The cancer patient receiving chemotherapy is worried about alopecia. The nurse is being supportive by stating:
1. "Just plan to get a hair piece. They look natural."
2. "That's one of the things you have to accept."
3. "Alopecia is actually very rare among cancer patients."
4. "Your hair will grow back after the chemo."

Answer: 4. "Your hair will grow back after the chemo."

Rationale: Hair loss is temporary during chemotherapy.

Nursing process: Intervention

Client need: Physiological integrity

Clinical skill level: 2

■ The nurse teaches a client that the following changes in a mole should be reported to the physician:
1. Growth of hair inside a mole
2. Development of solid light brown color
3. Development of uneven pigmentation with purplish color
4. Slow growth in size of any mole

Answer: 3. Development of uneven pigmentation with purplish color

Rationale: A significant change in pigmentation, including the presence of a purplish color, indicates that abnormal cells are present.

Nursing process: Assessment

Client need: Health promotion and maintenance

Clinical skill level: 2

■ Which skin tumor is most highly malignant?
1. Keratoses
2. Melanoma
3. Basal cell carcinoma
4. Squamous cell carcinoma

Answer: 2. Melanoma

Rationale: Melanoma has a poor prognosis unless treated early. Other skin malignancies have high cure rates even when diagnosed in an advanced stage.

Nursing process: Assessment

Client need: Physiological integrity

Clinical skill level: 1

HEMORRHAGE

DEFINITION
The loss of more than 500 cc of blood. The loss may be external or internal.

PATHOPHYSIOLOGY
Hemorrhage is classified:
- Class I: Blood loss of 750 ml
- Class II: Blood loss of 1,000 ml
- Class III: Blood loss of 1,500 ml
- Class IV: Blood loss of 2,000 ml

ASSOCIATED MEDICAL CONDITIONS
- Hypovolemic shock
- Intracranial hemorrhage
- Esophageal varies
- Subarachnoid hemorrhage

ASSESSMENT
- Pallor skin color
- Tachycardia
- Increasing/gasping respirations
- Thirst
- Cyanosis
- Black, tarry stool (internal)
- Pain in area of bleeding
- Vital signs every 15 minutes
- Cold, moist skin
- Hypotension
- Neurological signs every 15 minutes
- Drop in temperature
- Inspect wound
- Fever (internal hemorrhage)
- Restlessness/apprehension

CLIENT NEED
Physiological integrity

NURSING INTERVENTIONS
- Stop bleeding, if possible
- Administer blood
- Monitor for hypovolemic shock
- Administer IV fluids (use 14, 16, 18 gauge needles)
- Administer oxygen
- Keep warm with hyperthermia blankets

MEDICAL INTERVENTIONS
- Class I: Ringer's lactate (2L)
- Class II: Ringer's lactate (3-4L)
- Class III: Whole blood or RBCs
- Class IV: Combination of blood products and colloid fluids
- Antishock (MAST) trousers

ASSOCIATED NURSING DIAGNOSES
- Cardiac output, decreased
- Anxiety
- Fear
- Post-trauma response
- Tissue perfusion, altered (peripheral)
- Activity intolerance, high risk for
- Fatigue
- Fluid volume deficit
- Powerlessness

STUDY QUESTIONS

■ The nursing assessment reads: Subjective data: "exploding" headache, photophobia, nausea. Objective data: Extreme neck rigidity. The nurse prepares to treat this patient for:
1. Subdural hematoma
2. Cerebrovascular accident
3. Cerebral aneurysm
4. Subarachnoid hemorrhage

Answer: 4. Subarachnoid hemorrhage

Rationale: A subarachnoid hemorrhage is most commonly caused by the rupture of an intracranial aneurysm.

Nursing process: Assessment

Client need: Physiological integrity

Clinical skill level: 3

■ What diagnostic test is ordered when an intracranial hemorrhage is suspected?
1. Arteriogram
2. Brain scan
3. Bone scan
4. Cardiogram

Answer: 2. Brain scan

Rationale: A brain scan will indicate the location of bleeding in the brain.

Nursing process: Assessment

Client need: Physiological integrity

Clinical skill level: 2

■ The patient with an intracerebral hemorrhage is complaining of constipation. The nurse would prepare to administer:
1. A laxative
2. An enema
3. A stool softener
4. A slow enema

Answer: 3. A stool softener

Rationale: The valsalva maneuver, which is frequently used when a patient is straining at the stool, causes increased intracranial pressure and should be avoided in patients with neuro and cardiac diagnoses.

Nursing process: Intervention

Client need: Physiological integrity

Clinical skill level: 2

■ The nurse assesses signs of hemorrhage due to portal hypertension and notifies the physician. She prepares to administer:
1. Whole blood
2. Plasma protein
3. Vitamin A IM
4. Vitamin K IM

Answer: 4. Vitamin K IM

Rationale: Because this patient often suffers nutritional deficiencies, lack of vitamin K may cause a problem with blood clotting. The physician may order fresh frozen plasma or RBCs.

Nursing process: Intervention

Client need: Physiological integrity

Clinical skill level: 3

■ During the immediate post-operative period, the priority nursing assessment involves the detection of:
1. Infection
2. Sutures
3. Hemorrhage
4. Dressing

Answer: 3. Hemorrhage

Rationale: The post-operative patient is at greatest danger of hemorrhage within the first four hours following surgery.

Nursing process: Assessment

Client need: Physiological integrity

Clinical skill level: 2

■ A patient is scheduled for a liver biopsy. Which medication could contribute to a complication of the biopsy?
1. Zantac
2. Xylocaine
3. Aspirin
4. Morphine

Answer: 3. Aspirin

Rationale: The liver is highly vascular and hemorrhage is a significant threat following a biopsy. Aspirin interferes with platelet aggregation and increases risk of bleeding.

Nursing process: Evaluation

Client need: Physiological integrity

Clinical skill level: 2

HYPOVOLEMIC SHOCK

DEFINITION
A state of shock caused by massive fluid loss, most commonly hemorrhage.

PATHOPHYSIOLOGY
When blood volume is reduced by external blood loss through hemorrhage or loss of fluids, or internal transfer of blood to locations where it cannot circulate through relative hypovolemia in which the arterial blood vessels dilate and the blood volume is not great enough to fill the vascular system, the patient will go into hypovolemic shock.

ASSOCIATED MEDICAL CONDITIONS
- Renal disease
- Trauma with dramatic blood loss

ASSESSMENT
- Level of consciousness
- Monitor respiratory status
- Monitor peripheral pulses
- Monitor blood pressure
- Monitor breath sounds, especially crackles, when large amounts of IV fluids are being administered
- Patent airway
- Monitor ECG
- Monitor neurological status
- Monitor urine output

CLIENT NEED
Physiological integrity

NURSING INTERVENTIONS
- Maintain airway
- Strict I&O
- Administer O_2
- Administer IV fluids

- Observe bowel sounds
- MAST (antishock trousers)
- Keep patient warm
- Administer Ringer's lactate

ASSOCIATED NURSING DIAGNOSES
- Anxiety
- Cardiac output, decreased
- Fear
- Post-trauma response
- Tissue perfusion, altered (peripheral)
- Fatigue
- Activity intolerance, high risk for
- Fluid volume deficit
- Powerlessness

STUDY QUESTIONS

1. When a patient is suffering hypovolemic shock, the nurse prepares to administer:
   1. $D_{50}W$
   2. Normal saline
   3. Whole blood
   4. Ringer's lactate

   Answer: 4. Ringer's lactate

   Rationale: Lactated Ringer's will most likely be prescribed because it most closely resembles the composition of extracellular fluid. An isotonic solution such as normal saline might cause fluid overload.

   Nursing process: Intervention
   Client need: Physiological integrity

   Clinical skill level: 3

- The nurse carefully monitors the hypovolemic patient for signs of shock. What changes in vital signs will signal this complication?
    1. Decreasing blood pressure, decreasing pulse
    2. Decreasing blood pressure, increasing pulse
    3. Increasing blood pressure, increasing pulse
    4. Increasing blood pressure, decreasing pulse

    Answer: 2. Decreasing blood pressure, increasing pulse

    Rationale: The early signs of shock that are reflected in the vital signs are a drop in blood pressure and increase in pulse. Respirations also increase.

    Nursing process: Assessment

    Client need: Physiological integrity

    Level of clinical skill: 3

- Once the nurse evaluates that the patient is going into hypovolemic shock, what is the priority nursing action (provided there is an order for all of the following)?
    1. Check vital signs every five minutes
    2. Administer IV fluid stat
    3. Administer epinephrine stat
    4. Administer lidocaine IV stat

    Answer: 2. Administer IV fluid stat

    Rationale: The first measure instituted in most patients with shock is to replace fluids. At the onset of shock, the peripheral circulation diminishes as vessels constrict, and fluids help raise the circulatory volume and blood pressure.

    Nursing process: Intervention

    Client need: Physiological integrity

    Level of clinical skill: 4

INFORMED CONSENT

DEFINITION
Written permission that is signed by the patient after the patient has been freely informed regarding the scheduled procedure or surgery.

PATHOPHYSIOLOGY
Not applicable

ASSOCIATED MEDICAL CONDITIONS
- Surgery
- Radiation or cobalt therapy
- Chemotherapy
- Any invasive procedure
- Psychotropic medications

ASSESSMENT
- Does the patient ask questions that indicate lack of knowledge regarding the procedure or surgery?
- Has the patient been informed of the procedure or surgery?
- Does the patient make knowledgeable comments regarding the procedure or surgery?
- Does the patient voice a lack of knowledge regarding the outcome or prognosis of the procedure or surgery?

CLIENT NEED
Physiological integrity

NURSING INTERVENTIONS
- Explain procedure, if appropriate
- Allow patient time to ask questions

- Inform physician/surgeon if patient lacks basic knowledge of procedure or surgery
- Make sure consent has been signed before administering pre-op medication

PATIENT TEACHING
- Pain medication available
- Relaxation techniques that may be effective before procedure
- Approximate length of procedure

ASSOCIATED NURSING DIAGNOSES
- Anxiety
- Coping, ineffective individual
- Denial, ineffective
- Knowledge deficit

STUDY QUESTIONS

■ Which one of the following would constitute an invalid consent for surgery?
1. Signature obtained within 5 minutes after pre-operative medication administered
2. Making a mark of X in place of a signature
3. A 16-year-old married student receiving financial support
4. Consent heard by two persons per phone for a minor

Answer: 1. Signature obtained within 5 minutes after pre-operative medication administered

Rationale: The patient is not considered fully competent to make a decision to have surgery after the administration of the preoperative medications, which is often a narcotic.

Nursing process: Evaluation

Client need: Safe, effective care environment

Clinical skill level: 2

- The nurse is asked to get the patient to sign an informed consent form the day before surgery. The nurse recognizes her legal responsibility in regards to this legal document is:
    1. Witnessing the patient sign the form
    2. Assessing patient's knowledge about procedure
    3. Making sure that the patient knows the risks
    4. Asking a relative to co-sign as a witness

    Answer: 1. Witnessing the patient sign the form

    Rationale: The nurse's responsibility regarding informed consent is witnessing the patient's signature. It is the physician's responsibility to inform the patient of the procedure or surgery, including the potential side effects and risks. The nurse, however, does have the responsibility to contact the physician if the patient indicates that they lack some knowledge of the procedure or the potential outcome.

    Nursing process: Intervention

    Client need: Safe, effective care environment

    Level of clinical skill: 2

LEAD POISONING

DEFINITION
A toxic level of lead in the blood. Lead is found in paint and water in lead pipes.

PATHOPHYSIOLOGY
Lead-poisoning is the leading heavy metal intoxication in the United States. Sources include tenements where the walls are chipping and peeling with lead paint, industries where lead is processed, storage batteries, spray paints, improperly fired ceramics, and moonshine whiskey distilled in automobile radiators. When lead is consumed it enters the bloodstream.

ASSOCIATED MEDICAL CONDITIONS
- Renal failure
- Abdominal distress
- Depression
- Blood dyscarias

ASSESSMENT
- Colic
- Peripheral neuritis
- Lead in urine
- Anemia
- Encephalopathy
- Lead in blood

CLIENT NEED
Physiological integrity

NURSING INTERVENTIONS
- Administer medications prescribed
- Monitor fluid balance to ensure excretion of lead. Offer large amounts of milk to help deposit lead from blood stream into bone.

MEDICAL INTERVENTIONS
- Prescribe dimercaprol
- Prescribe calcium disodium Versenate
- Prescribe Penicillamine

PATIENT TEACHING
- No cure is available; emphasis is on palliative care
- Seek support group or psychological counseling to deal with psychological aspects of disease process
- Identify source of lead and remove from environment
-

ASSOCIATED NURSING DIAGNOSES
- Anxiety
- Fluid volume deficit
- Post-trauma response
- Role performance, altered
- Coping, ineffective individual
- Fear
- Knowledge deficit
- Poisoning, high risk for
- Tissue perfusion, altered (gastrointestinal, peripheral)

STUDY QUESTIONS

■ In patient teaching, the nurse stresses regular checkups even after the source of lead poisoning has been eliminated. The rationale for this is that lead poisoning eventually affects the:
1. Heart failure
2. Fluid balance
3. Endocrine system
4. Nervous system

Answer: 4. Nervous system

Rationale: Because lead usually cannot be completely flushed out of the system, side effects could occur for several years.

Nursing process: Intervention

Client need: Physiological integrity

Clinical skill level: 3

■ In forcing fluids to the patient with lead poisoning, the nurse encourages the patient to drink a lot of:
1. Water
2. Milk
3. Fruit juice
4. Carrot juice

Answer: 2. Milk

Rationale: Milk will combine with circulating lead, and it becomes a lead salt and is then deposited in the bone, out of the blood circulation.

Nursing process: Intervention

Client need: Physiological integrity

Clinical skill level: 4

MALIGNANT HYPERTHERMIA

DEFINITION
A genetic muscle disorder that is triggered by anesthesia and characterized by muscle contractions. If untreated, the hyperthermia is potentially fatal.

PATHOPHYSIOLOGY
The pathophysiology of this disorder occurs at the cellular level. In malignant hyperthermia, anesthetic agents trigger a sudden increase of calcium ions within the muscle cell which, in turn, starts a series of biochemical reactions that elevate the metabolic rate and create the clinical symptoms of constant muscle contraction or rigidity, hyperthermia and CNS damage. The condition may occur within 30 minutes of administration of anesthesia or happen hours following surgery.

ASSESSMENT
- Fever (as high as 104°F)
- Diaphoresis
- Rigidity, especially in the jaw (early sign)
- Hypotension
- Oliguria
- Cyanosis/mottling of skin
- Identify at-risk patients
- Tetany
- Tachycardia (over 150/min.—an early sign)
- Decreasing cardiac output
- Cardiac arrest
- Ventricular dysrhythmia

CLIENT NEED
Physiological integrity

NURSING INTERVENTIONS
- Early detection
- Accurate history of death of any family members during or after surgery

- History of muscle weakness
- Hyperventilate with 100% O$_2$
- History of muscle cramps

- Lavage of stomach/colon with iced saline
- Application of cool packs or hyperthermia blanket
- Administer sodium bicarbonate IV

MEDICAL INTERVENTIONS
- Prompt DC of anesthesia
- Prescribe Dantrolene (muscle relaxant) (1mg/kg body weight up to 10 mg 1 kg)

PATIENT TEACHING
- Alert surgeon to family history of death of febrile response during or following surgery

ASSOCIATED NURSING DIAGNOSES
- Fear
- Gas exchange, impaired
- Body temperature, high risk for altered
- Cardiac output, decreased
- Hyperthermia
- Tissue perfusion, altered

STUDY QUESTION

■ In assessing a patient for malignant hyperthermia, the first indication prior to surgery that the patient is at risk is:
1. Higher than normal body temperature
2. Small, wasting muscle tone
3. Excessive restlessness related to surgery
4. A family history of febrile reaction during surgery

Answer: 4. A family history of febrile reaction during surgery

Rationale: Malignant hyperthermia is an inherited disorder in which the person's genetic makeup predisposes them to this dramatic side effect of anesthesia.

Nursing process: Assessment

Client need: Physiological integrity

Clinical skill level: 3

PAIN

DEFINITION
Pain is whatever the patient says that it is. It is a subjective, often emotional experience that may or may not have an obvious physiological base.

PATHOPHYSIOLOGY
Nerve endings called nociceptors are stimulated by a stimuli that may cause tissue damage. The stimuli is transmitted via the spinal cord to the brain where the stimuli is perceived as painful. Chronic pain is the same pain in approximately the same location lasting for six months or more.

ASSESSMENT
- Location of the pain; ask patient to point with index finger
- Quality of pain such as burning, stabbing sharp
- Depression that may be associated with chronic pain
- Intensity of pain, usually on a scale of 1-5 or 1-10. Duration, or length of time the pain has persisted.
- Radiation of pain to another site
- Assess patient's coping strategies in dealing with the pain

CLIENT NEED
Physiological integrity

INTERVENTION
- Remove the stimuli causing pain, if possible
- Teach relaxation techniques
- Promote sleep and rest
- Assist patient in reducing anxiety
- Administer pain medications as prescribed
- Provide optimal nutritional intake
- Teach distraction techniques
- Evaluate response to pain medications

PATIENT TEACHING

- Teach self-care techniques for relieving pain, such as guided imagery, relaxation
- Teach how to use pain medication for optimal relief, such as taking medications before pain becomes intense

ASSOCIATED NURSING DIAGNOSES

- Anxiety
- Communication, impaired verbal
- Fear
- Knowledge deficit
- Pain
- Powerlessness
- Fatigue
- Disuse syndrome, high risk for
- Injury, high risk for
- Noncompliance
- Pain, chronic
- Social interaction, impaired

STUDY QUESTIONS

■ A patient is 8 hours post-op and complaining of moderate pain at the abdominal incision site. The blood pressure is slightly elevated, 130/80. The pain medication ordered is not due for another hour. Which intervention is appropriate?
1. Calmly explain that he must wait 4 hours between injections
2. Reposition and offer a back rub
3. Recheck dressing and retake blood pressure
4. Call the doctor stat and get another medication order

Answer: 2. Reposition and offer a back rub

Rationale: The best nursing intervention is to assist the patient in relaxation and distraction as a way to cope with moderate pain. It is, however, the responsibility of the nurse to report to the physician when a pain medication is not effectively relieving pain.

Nursing process: Intervention

Client need: Physiological integrity

Clinical skill level: 2

- Endorphins are the body's natural opiate-like substances that transmit and inhibit painful stimuli. In which personality are endorphins higher?
    1. The depressed person who takes medication
    2. The happy person who laughs a lot
    3. The anxious person who cries a lot
    4. The psychotic who sleeps 10-16 hours a day

    Answer: 2. The happy person who laughs a lot

    Rationale: Research shows that activities such as laughter, exercise, and an optimistic attitude enhance the secretion of endorphins.

    Nursing process: Assessment

    Client need: Physiological integrity

    Clinical skill level: 2

- When doing a pain assessment, the nurse should be alert to what the patient says. The patient in acute pain may not be able to describe the pain, and the nurse should be primarily concerned in assessing:
    1. The location and quality of pain
    2. The medication the physician should order
    3. Whether the pain has a real physiological basis
    4. The emotional and psychological responses to pain

    Answer: 1. The location and quality of pain

    Rationale: The kind of intervention required will depend upon these two characteristics of pain. For example, the nurse must make the decision whether or not to administer medication (if ordered) or to call the physician.

    Nursing process: Assessment

    Client need: Physiological integrity

    Clinical skill level: 2

■ To assess the quality of pain, the nurse would ask:
1. "Tell me what your pain feels like."
2. "Is your pain a crushing sensation?"
3. "How long have you had this pain?"
4. "Is it a sharp pain or dull pain?"

Answer: 1. "Tell me what your pain feels like."

Rationale: With this question the nurse is asking for a description without leading the patient. If the patient cannot describe the pain, then the nurse can give examples such as crushing, dull pressure, sharp or stabbing pain.

Nursing process: Assessment

Client need: Physiological integrity

Clinical skill level: 2

■ According to research, patients experience more pain during:
1. The day
2. The night
3. Visiting hours
4. Morning hours

Answer: 2. The night

Rationale: Although the reasons for this are inconclusive, more patients complain of pain at night. Perhaps the distractions of day-time activities is one reason.

Nursing process: Assessment

Client need: Physiological integrity

Clinical skill level: 1

■ The best assessment of pain can be determined when the patient:
1. Trembles as he speaks
2. Never moves his body
3. Clenches his teeth as he speaks
4. States he has pain

Answer: 4. States he has pain

Rationale: Because pain is subjective, the nurse must carefully assess what the patient says about the location, quality, and intensity of the pain and should never discount the presence of pain because the client does not manifest visible symptoms.

Nursing process: Assessment

Client need: Physiological integrity

Clinical skill level: 2

■ A nurse can prepare a patient for a painful experience such as surgery and invasive procedures by:
1. Telling the patient most pain is psychological
2. Explain the body's pain mechanism in detail
3. Tell the patient that complaining is childish
4. Teach the patient about pain and its relief

Answer: 4. Teach the patient about pain and its relief

Rationale: Teaching the patient about pain medications and techniques to relieve pain decreases anxiety, thus giving the patient more of a sense of control over the pain.

Nursing process: Intervention

Client need: Physiological integrity

Clinical skill level: 2

■ Pain that arises from the internal organs is called:
1. Cultaneous
2. Visceral
3. Radiating
4. Phantom

Answer: 2. Visceral

Rationale: Visceral implies internal organs and usually refers to abdominal pain.

Nursing process: Assessment

Client need: Physiological integrity

Clinical skill level: 1

■ A 34-year-old man suffered a traumatic amputation of his right foot in a car accident. He is receiving meperidine (Demerol) 100 mg IM and acetaminophen (Tylenol) gr 10 PO every 3 hours for pain. He complains of a burning sensation in the right foot. The nurse explains:
1. Phantom pain is a phenomenon not clearly understood
2. This is not real because the foot was amputated
3. His regular medication should relieve the pain
4. This phantom pain will disappear in about 6 months

Answer: 1. Phantom pain is a phenomenon not clearly understood

Rationale: Phantom pain is real, and should be treated as any other pain.

Nursing process: Intervention

Client need: Physiological integrity

Clinical skill level: 2

- One afternoon when the patient appears uncomfortable, the nurse asks if he wants his pain medication. He replies, "No, I'll just wait until it gets really bad." The nurse responds:
  1. "Okay, let me know when you're ready"
  2. "If you let the pain become severe, the medication will not work as well."
  3. "I respect you for handling pain the way you do."
  4. "Good, I'm glad you're concerned about getting addicted."

  Answer: 2. "If you let the pain become severe, the medication will not work as well."

  Rationale: Pain medication is most effective when administered as soon as possible. When the pain is severe, it takes more medication over a longer period of time to control it.

  Nursing process: Intervention

  Client need: Physiological integrity

  Clinical skill level: 2

- Patient-controlled analgesia (PCA) is a method by which the patient administers pain medication to himself. Studies show patients using PCA:
  1. Take more medication than necessary
  2. Take less medication, generally
  3. Take pain medication when pain is not severe
  4. Take pain medication too often

  Answer: 2. Take less medication, generally

  Rationale: When the patient is in control of the administration of medication, anxiety is decreased. Research shows this decreases the need for more medication.

  Nursing process: Evaluation

  Client need: Physiological integrity

  Clinical skill level: 2

■ Placebos are administered by the nurse when:
  1. The patient is addicted to drugs
  2. The patient is faking pain to get drugs
  3. The physician orders this kind of drug
  4. The patient exhibits a typical response to pain

  Answer: 3. The physician orders this kind of drug
  Rationale: Placebos are prescribed just as any other medication.
  Nursing process: Intervention
  Client need: Physiological integrity

  Clinical skill level: 2

■ The nurse administers pain medication IM and she knows it should be effective:
  1. Immediately
  2. In 3-5 minutes
  3. In 15-20 minutes
  4. Over a period of an hour

  Answer: 3. In 15-20 minutes
  Rationale: IM medications are absorbed into the bloodstream and is effective in 15-20 minutes.
  Nursing process: Outcome criteria
  Client need: Physiological integrity

  Clinical skill level: 2

- Pain is a subjective assessment. For the nurse planning care for the patient in pain, this means:
    1. Pain depends upon the physical source
    2. Pain must be physical to justify medication
    3. The nurse must be able to justify the pain
    4. Pain is whatever the patient says that it is

    Answer: 4. Pain is whatever the patient says that it is

    Rationale: The nurse must carefully assess how the patient describes pain, and treat the symptom accordingly.

    Nursing process: Assessment

    Client need: Physiological integrity

    Clinical skill level: 2

SHOCK

DEFINITION

Shock is an insufficient tissue perfusion resulting from lack of sufficient oxygen to the cells. Because of the lack of proper oxygenation, cells do not metabolise properly, and waste products accumulate

Classifications of shock include:
- Hypovolemic
- Cardiogenic
- Neurogenic
- Septic

PATHOPHYSIOLOGY

During shock, epinephrine and norepinephrine levels are incr eased and work to constrict arterioles in the skin, subcutaneous tissue, and kidneys while dilating arterioles of skeletal muscles and liver. Cardiac output increases, as does plasma level of glococorticoids. Glycogen is released to supply energy and endorphins are released to lower blood pressure. Because of the decrease in cardiac output and the lack of sufficient insulin, oxygen utilization also decreases.

MOST COMMON MEDICAL CONDITIONS

- Hemorrhage
- Poisoning
- Myocardial infarction
- Renal failure

ASSESSMENT

Classical signs/symptoms:
- Cool, moist skin
- Hyperventilation
- Increasing, weak, thready pulse
- Dropping blood pressure
- Pallor
- Cyanosis (first sign around lips, tongue, gums)
- Progressively decreasing pulse pressure
- Concentrated urine output< 30 ml/hr

Follow-up assessment:
- CVP
- Serum lactate levels ("the higher the level, the greater the oxygen need")
- LOC—as shock progresses the patient will deteriorate into coma
- ABGs
- Hematocrit (results help to determine what kind of fluid replacement required)

NURSING INTERVENTIONS
- Encourage deep breathing to promote cardiopulmonary function.
- Administer blood, blood products as ordered
- Quiet environment to decrease anxiety
- Control pain (especially in MI; cardiogenic shock)
- Administer IV fluids
- Monitor VS and be alert for ↑ pulse, ↑ respirations, and ↓ blood pressure
- Keep patient warm (avoid overheating that might further dilate vessels)
- Measure/estimate blood loss if indicated (Hemorrhage is 500 ml)
- Administer narcotics judiciously
- Place in supine to facilitate circulation. Legs should be elevated 20-30°
- Turn patient every 2 hours

MEDICAL INTERVENTIONS
- Intropin, Levophed, and Neo-Synephrine are used as vasoconstrictors which elevate blood pressure and increase blood flow to the brain and heart.
- Amrinone, dobutamine, and Nipride dilate vessels, improve capillary flow, tissue perfusion and cellular metabolism.
- Antibiotics, Heparin, Calcium.

PATIENT TEACHING

- Report feelings of anxiety, restlessness
- Deep breathing to decrease anxiety

ASSOCIATED NURSING DIAGNOSES

- Decreased cardiac output
- Injury, high risk for
- Anxiety
- Tissue perfusion, altered: cerebral, cardiopulmonary, rental, gastrointestinal, peripheral
- Breathing pattern, ineffective
- Fluid volume deficit
- Role performance, altered

STUDY QUESTIONS

■ The nurse assesses that an increase in pulse rate is a warning sign of:
1. Dystonia
2. Shock
3. Dysrhythmias
4. Drug toxicity

Answer: 2. Shock

Rationale: Signs of shock are falling blood pressure, increasing pulse and respirations.

Nursing process: Assessment

Client need: Physiological integrity

Clinical skill level: 2

■ The nurse assesses the patient who is going into shock. What changes in vital signs are assessed?
1. Decreasing blood pressure, decreasing pulse
2. Decreasing blood pressure, increasing pulse
3. Increasing blood pressure, increasing pulse
4. Increasing blood pressure, decreasing pulse

Answer: 2. Decreasing blood pressure, increasing pulse

Rationale: In the early stages of shock the nurse will observe falling blood pressure, increasing pulse and increasing respirations.

Nursing process: Evaluation

Client need: Physiological integrity

Clinical skill level: 2

■ This is the nursing assessment of a post-operative patient's blood pressure: 120/70 at 1 a.m., 100/70 at 10:15 a.m., and 90/60 at 10:25 a.m. These readings indicate that the patient:
1. Is going into shock
2. Is responding favorably
3. Is normally hypotensive
4. Is getting too much IV fluid

Answer: 1. Is going into shock

Rationale: A steady drop in blood pressure is a sign of impending shock. This patient may be hemorrhaging.

Nursing process: Assessment

Client need: Physiological integrity

Clinical skill level: 3

■ A patient's blood culture is positive for gram negative bacteria. Further assessment shows tachycardia (120/min) and hypotension. These signs are indicative of:
1. Cariogenic shock
2. Hypovolemic shock
3. Septic shock
4. Vasogenic shock

Answer: 3. Septic shock

Rationale: In an attempt to compensate, cardiac output will increase and the release of histamine and increasing endorphin levels causes vasodilation. This process produces the hypotension.

Nursing process: Evaluation

Client need: Physiological integrity

Clinical skill level: 4

■ The ER nurse notifies the floor nurse that the patient being transferred for admission to the hospital is "shocky." The nurse will closely monitor for:
1. Increased blood pressure and decreases pulse
2. Increased pulse and decreased respiratory
3. Decreased respiratory and increased blood pressure
4. Increased respirations and decreased blood pressure

Answer: 4. Increased respirations and decreased blood pressure

Rationale: The signs of shock are increasing respirations, increasing pulse, and falling blood pressure.

Nursing process: Assessment

Client need: Physiological integrity

Clinical skill level: 3

METABOLIC ALKALOSIS

DEFINITION
Metabolic alkalosis is a disturbance resulting from a high plasma bicarbonate accumulation and an abnormal loss of acid.

PATHOPHYSIOLOGY
Hypokalemia is the most common cause of metabolic alkalosis; however, the disorder can also be caused by the loss of hydrogen and chloride ions through vomiting or gastric suction. When the body is deficient in potassium, H+ is secreted into the urine in exchange for sodium. This process causes reabsorption of bicarbonate.

ASSOCIATED MEDICAL CONDITIONS
- Coma resulting from severe, untreated alkalosis
- Hypokalemia

ASSESSMENT
- s/s hyperkalemia: weakness, tetany,
- s/s of phlebitis, especially if potassium is being administered
- Electrolyte imbalance
- I & O
- Respirations, usually decreased to compensate
- s/s hypokalemia: hypotension, tachycardia
- Seizures

CLIENT NEED
Physiological integrity

NURSING INTERVENTIONS
- Allen test
- Positioning
- Pulmonary hygiene
- Hydration

MEDICAL INTERVENTIONS
- Sodium chloride fluids are administered to restore normal fluid volume.
- Ringer's solution
- Intravenous administration of HCl or ammonium chloride or arginine hydrochloride may be used.

PATIENT TEACHING
- Identify those prescriptions which cause imbalances
- Take prescribed medications
- Learn to take own pulse and check for signs of imbalances
- Choose foods and beverages which will prevent electrolyte imbalance

ASSOCIATED NURSING DIAGNOSES
- Breathing pattern, ineffective
- Fear
- Ventilation, inability to sustain spontaneous
- Tissue perfusion, altered: peripheral
- Fatigue

Unit 13

COMPREHENSIVE TEST

- General test questions to prepare the student for the NCLEX

❏ A patient is diagnosed with end-stage syphilis. What signs and symptoms are associated with this condition?
1. Severe headaches and confusion
2. Paralysis in all extremities
3. Blindness and paralysis
4. Slapping gait and blindness

Answer: 4. Slapping gait and blindness

Rationale: In the end stages of syphilis, degeneration in the dorsal root causes shrinkage and fibrosis in the spinal cord that produces CNS damage.

Nursing process: Assessment

Client need: Physiological integrity

| Clinical skill level: 2 |

❏ The nurse suspects the cardiac surgery patient has a pneumothorax. The cardiac sign of this complication is:
1. Crackles
2. Rhonchi
3. Tracheobronchial secretions
4. Absent breath sounds

Answer: 4. Absent breath sounds

Rationale: One of the first signs of pneumothorax is decreasing or absent breath sounds.

Nursing process: Assessment

Client need: Physiological integrity

| Clinical skill level: 3 |

❏ Prolonged immobility can cause which electrolyte imbalance?
   1. Hyperkalemia
   2. Hypokalemia
   3. Hypercalcemia
   4. Hypocalcemia

   Answer: 3. Hypercalcemia

   Rationale: With extended periods of immobility, calcium moves out of the bone and into the bloodstream.

   Nursing process: Evaluation

   Client need: Physiological integrity

   Clinical skill level: 4

❏ If the patient is experiencing hyperkalemia, the nurse should prepare to administer:
   1. Kayexalate
   2. KCL
   3. Digitalis
   4. Diuretics

   Answer: 1. Kayexalate

   Rationale: Sodium polystyrene sulfonate (Kayexalate) is an iron-exchange resin that binds potassium and promotes potassium excretion through the intestines.

   Nursing process: Intervention

   Client need: Physiological integrity

   Clinical skill level: 3

❏ Planning care for the cardiac surgery patient focuses on prevention of the postcardiotomy syndrome, which may be caused by anxiety, sensory overload, or sleep deprivation. The nurse plan should emphasize:
1. Regular meals
2. Regular medication
3. Relaxation techniques
4. Uninterrupted sleep

Answer: 4. Uninterrupted sleep

Rationale: Interrupted sleep cycles cause sleep deprivation and disorientation. The length of sleep cycles vary from 50 to 120 minutes, with each successive cycle growing shorter.

Nursing process: Outcome criteria

Client need: Physiological integrity

Clinical skill level: 3

❏ The physician writes an order for Buerger-Allen exercises. These are active postural exercises recommended to reverse:
1. Venous obstruction
2. Arterial insufficiency
3. Venous insufficiency
4. Thrombotic occlusions

Answer: 2. Arterial insufficiency

Rationale: This is a series of exercises that involve the patient lying supine with legs elevated for at least three minutes, then sitting up with legs dependent for three minutes, and then lying flat with legs horizontal with the body for at least five minutes.

Nursing process: Outcome criteria

Client need: Physiological integrity

Clinical skill level: 3

❏ The patient using crutches should be taught at least two crutch gaits to relieve fatigue. The nurse teaches the patient that the rationale for this is:
1. The patient will enjoy a variety of gaits
2. One gait may be too limiting in mobility
3. Gaits differ as extremity heals
4. Each gait uses different muscles

Answer: 4. Each gait uses different muscles

Rationale: The patient should be taught to vary crutch gaits because if one group of muscles is forced to sustain steady contraction, circulation may be impaired.

Nursing process: Intervention

Client need: Physiological integrity

Clinical skill level: 2

❏ In teaching the patient to use different crutch gaits, the nurse uses the theory that all gaits are based on:
1. The nature of the disability
2. The tripod position
3. The height of the patient
4. The age of the patient

Answer: 2. The tripod position

Rationale: The tripod position is assumed when the crutches are about 8 to 10 inches in front and to the side of the patient's toes. The position provides for maximum stability.

Nursing process: Intervention

Client need: Physiological integrity

Clinical skill level: 3

❏ Lab results show the patient has high potassium levels in the blood. The nurse is aware that the major complication of hyperkalemia is:
1. Associated sodium excess
2. Hyperventilation and acidosis
3. Overstimulation of nerve tissue
4. Overstimulation of cardiac muscle

Answer: 4. Overstimulation of cardiac muscle

Rationale: The signs and symptoms of hyperkalemia are irritability, diarrhea, and ECG changes.

Nursing process: Assessment

Client need: Physiological integrity

Clinical skill level: 3

❏ The early signs the nurse must assess in monitoring for hypokalemia is:
1. Muscle spasm, nausea
2. Restlessness, irritability
3. Muscle weakness, apathy
4. Paralysis associated with pain

Answer: 3. Muscle weakness, apathy

Rationale: Muscle weakness and apathy are the result of decreased muscular stimulation by the nervous system. Other signs of hypokalemia are diminished reflexes, weak pulse and shallow respirations.

Nursing process: Assessment

Client need: Physiological integrity

Clinical skill level: 3

❏ In assessing the patient suspected of having a fluid and electrolyte imbalance, the nurse is aware that the major cation that regulates intracellular osmolality is:
1. Sodium
2. Chloride
3. Magnesium
4. Potassium

Answer: 4. Potassium

Rationale: Sodium and potassium are the major cations that regulate fluid balance in the body. Sodium is found primarily in extracellular fluid.

Nursing process: Assessment

Client need: Physiological integrity

Clinical skill level: 2

❏ Another important factor in assessing this patient is that the regulator of extracellular osmolality is:
1. Sodium
2. Calcium
3. Potassium
4. Magnesium

Answer: 1. Sodium

Rationale: Sodium regulates the osmotic pressure of extracellular fluid as well as maintaining the acid-base balance in the body.

Nursing process: Assessment

Client need: Physiological integrity

Clinical skill level: 2

❑ The patient with sodium imbalance must be assessed for what other electrolyte imbalance?
1. Chloride
2. Magnesium
3. Calcium
4. Potassium

Answer: 4. Potassium

Rationale: Sodium and potassium work together, constantly moving in and out of cells, propelled by sodium-potassium pumps.

Nursing process: Assessment

Client need: Physiological integrity

Clinical skill level: 2

❑ A patient has diarrhea for 6 days. In reviewing the laboratory tests, the nurse should assess the serum level of:
1. Calcium chloride
2. Creatinine
3. Potassium
4. Blood urea nitrogen

Answer: 3. Potassium

Rationale: The most common electrolyte imbalance related to diarrhea is hypokalemia.

Nursing process: Evaluation

Client need: Physiological integrity

Clinical skill level: 3

❏ The patient with nasogastric suction is most likely to experience which electrolyte imbalance?
   1. Hypokalemia
   2. Hypomagnesemia
   3. Hyponatremia
   4. Hypernatremia

   Answer: 1. Hypokalemia

   Rationale: Nasogastric suctioning draws out H^+ and Cl^- in the GI fluid that is being lost. Hypokalemia is the result of the metabolic alkalosis caused by the loss of acid.

   Nursing process: Assessment

   Client need: Physiological integrity

   Clinical skill level: 2

❏ When a patient is prescribed a diuretic, such as Lasix, careful assessment must be directed to:
   1. Pulse rate
   2. Pulse pressure
   3. Blood pressure
   4. Electrolyte imbalance

   Answer: 4. Electrolyte imbalance

   Rationale: Loop diuretics cause an increased excretion of potassium. Hypokalemia is a frequent side effect.

   Nursing process: Assessment

   Client need: Physiological integrity

   Clinical skill level: 2

❏ A trauma patient has received multiple blood transfusions over the past 48 hours. Which electrolyte imbalance should be assessed?
1. Hyperkalemia
2. Hypocalcemia
3. Hyperglycemia
4. Hyponatremia

Answer: 1. Hyperkalemia
Rationale: Stored blood has increased levels of potassium. Since the higher potassium level is due to the deterioration of red blood cells, the longer the blood is stored, the higher the potassium levels.
Nursing process: Assessment
Client need: Physiological integrity

Clinical skill level: 3

❏ The patient is started on furosemide (Lasix), a loop diuretic. A major concern in the administration of diuretics is the likelihood of:
1. Hypokalemia
2. Hyponatremia
3. Hypocalcemia
4. Hypomagnesium

Answer: 1. Hypokalemia
Rationale: Loop diuretics wash potassium out of the body, often causing hypokalemia.
Nursing process: Outcome criteria
Client need: Physiological integrity

Clinical skill level: 3

❏   The physician orders enemas until clear. The nurse should restrict the total to three enemas because there is an electrolyte imbalance associated with excessive enemas. Which imbalance is of most concern?
    1. Hypercalcemia
    2. Hypocalcemia
    3. Hyperkalemia
    4. Hypokalemia

    Answer: 4. Hypokalemia

    Rationale: Enemas will wash potassium out of the body, via osmosis and more than three enemas may cause low potassium depending upon the general condition of the patient.

    Nursing process: Assessment

    Client need: Physiological integrity

    Clinical skill level: 3

❏   In teaching the patient using a walker, the nurse evaluates which as correct positioning?
    1. Elbows held out straight
    2. Elbows flexed at 20-30 degree angle
    3. Elbows flexed at 60-80 degree angle
    4. Place hands loosely on side of walker

    Answer: 2. Elbows flexed at 20-30 degree angle

    Rationale: The patient should be taught to grip the walker firmly and walk into the walker. It is important that the elbows be slightly flexed to achieve balance.

    Nursing process: Intervention

    Client need: Physiological integrity

    Clinical skill level: 2

❑ A patient with a decubitus ulcer is ordered a special flotation mattress. The rationale for this is that a fluid-filled bed:
1. Automatically massages sensitive areas
2. Reduces shearing forces when lifted
3. Creates less pressure on susceptible body parts
4. Improves mobility when the patient turns in bed

Answer: 3. Creates less pressure on susceptible body parts

Rationale: The flotation mattress is based on Pascal's law which states that the weight of the body on a fluid mattress is evenly distributed over the entire body, thereby relieving pressure over the bony prominences.

Nursing process: Intervention

Client need: Physiological integrity

Clinical skill level: 2

❑ The physician orders a carminative enema of 30 ml of magnesium sulfate, 60 ml glycerin, and 90 ml warm water. The purpose of this enema is:
1. Cleanse prior to visualization
2. To relieve flatus
3. To draw fluid into intestine
4. Removing impaction

Answer: 2. To relieve flatus

Rationale: This 1-2-3 enema relieves flatus and constipation by intestinal mucosal irritation.

Nursing process: Outcome criteria

Client need: Physiological integrity

Clinical skill level: 2

❑ An isotonic enema of normal saline is contraindicated in a patient with:
1. Chronic constipation
2. Laxative abuse
3. Cardiac problems
4. Fecal impaction

Answer: 3. Cardiac problems

Rationale: Normal saline is retained in the intestine due to its osmotic effect, stimulates peristalsis by increasing bulk in the intestines.

Nursing process: Intervention

Client need: Physiological integrity

Clinical skill level: 3

❑ Following a laryngectomy, the optimal position is:
1. Low Fowler's
2. Semi-Fowler's
3. Supine
4. Recumbent

Answer: 2. Semi-Fowler's

Rationale: Respiratory excursion is promoted by positioning the patient so that the diaphragm can optimally expand.

Nursing process: Outcome criteria

Client need: Physiological integrity

Clinical skill level: 2

❏ Which assessment is the first indication that the post-laryngectomy patient is experiencing respiratory and/or circulatory difficulties?
1. Restlessness and apprehension
2. Increasing complaints of pain
3. Inability to communicate
4. Confusion and disorientation

Answer: 1. Restlessness and apprehension

Rationale: Other indicators that signal an airway problem are labored breathing and tachycardia.

Nursing process: Assessment

Client need: Physiological integrity

Clinical skill level: 3

❏ Following a thoracentesis, the nurse assesses a crackling sensation resembling crinkled paper upon palpation. The face, neck, and scrotum are particularly affected. This assessment is indicative of:
1. Pneumonia
2. Closed pneumothorax
3. Airway obstruction
4. Subcutaneous emphysema

Answer: 4. Subcutaneous emphysema

Rationale: During a thoracentesis, air from the pleural cavity infiltrates into the subcutaneous tissue, causing subcutaneous emphysema. This condition is usually not threatening unless it is left untreated and begins to affect vital organs, such as the trachea.

Nursing process: Assessment

Client need: Physiological integrity

Clinical skill level: 3

❏ The priority nursing intervention for a patient with subcutaneous emphysema is:
1. IV therapy
2. Narcotic administration
3. High concentrations of O_2
4. Turn, cough, deep breathe

Answer: 3. High concentrations of O_2

Rationale: The reabsorption of air in the subcutaneous tissues is enhanced because oxygen washes nitrogen out of the blood and this, in turn, enhances diffusion from subcutaneous tissues back into circulation.

Nursing process: Intervention

Client need: Physiological integrity

Clinical skill level: 3

❏ The first priority in cardiopulmonary resuscitation is:
1. Rescue breathing
2. Calling for help
3. Establishing airway
4. Cardiac compressions

Answer: 3. Establishing airway

Rationale: Airway is the priority intervention in any emergency. The head-tilt/chin-tilt maneuver is recommended to open airway quickly without risk of damage to the spinal cord.

Nursing process: Intervention

Client need: Physiological integrity

Clinical skill level: 2

❏ If the bag and mask technique is used during CPR, the ventilation rate is:
1. 9 breaths per minute
2. 10 breaths per minute
3. 12 breaths per minute
4. 16 breaths per minute

Answer: 3. 12 breaths per minute

Rationale: A rate of 12 beats per minute is within the normal respiratory rate, and should provide oxygenation needs until other emergency measures (such as mechanical ventilation) are in place or until the patient begins to breathe on his own.

Nursing process: Intervention

Client need: Physiological integrity

Clinical skill level: 2

❏ The two criteria that are essential when CPR is initiated are:
1. No heartbeat, no response
2. No help available, no response
3. No movement, no response
4. No respirations, no pulse

Answer: 4. No respirations, no pulse

Rationale: Breathlessness and pulselessness are the primary reasons that CPR is started. If there is either breath or pulse, other emergency measures are indicated

Nursing process: Assessment

Client need: Physiological integrity

Clinical skill level: 2

❏ The number of compressions required during CPR are:
1. 20/min
2. 40/min
3. 60/min
4. 80/min

Answer: 3. 60/min

Rationale: The regular compression and release rate required for adequate circulation is 60/minute.

Nursing process: Assessment

Client need: Physiological integrity

> Clinical skill level: 2

❏ In one-man CPR, the ventilation-compression ratio is:
1. 1 ventilation, 5 compressions
2. 2 ventilations, 10 compressions
3. 2 ventilations, 15 compressions
4. 4 ventilations, 15 compressions

Answer: 3. 2 ventilations, 15 compressions

Rationale: The American Heart Association recommends the 2-15 ratio for adequate oxygenation and circulation. The compression rate is 80-100 per minute.

Nursing process: Intervention

Client need: Physiological integrity

> Clinical skill level: 2

❏ In two-man CPR, the ventilation-compression ratio is:
1. 1 ventilation, 5 compressions
2. 1 ventilation, 10 compressions
3. 2 ventilations, 10 compressions
4. 2 ventilations, 15 compressions

Answer: 1. 1 ventilation, 5 compressions

Rationale: The ratio of 5-1 with a rate of 80-100 per minute. After 5 compressions the ventilator stops to allow for ventilation.

Nursing process: Intervention

Client need: Physiological integrity

Clinical skill level: 2

❏ During cardiopulmonary bypass surgery, the patient requires anticoagulation therapy. The nurse prepares to administer:
1. Coumadin
2. Heparin
3. Vitamin K
4. Streptokinase

Answer: 2. Heparin

Rationale: Anticoagulation therapy with Heparin is essential to prevent thrombus formation and the danger of embolus. Embolization is a more prominent threat during the time the blood comes into contact with the cardiopulmonary bypass circuit outside body circulation

Nursing process: Intervention

Client need: Physiological integrity

Clinical skill level: 3

❏ To reverse the effects of Heparin following bypass surgery, the nurse administers:
   1. Urokinase
   2. Warfarin Sodium
   3. Vitamin K
   4. Protamine sulfate

   Answer: 4. Protamine sulfate
   Rationale: The antagonist for Heparin is protamine sulfate and will quickly reverse the effects of heparin.
   Nursing process: Intervention
   Client need: Physiological integrity

   Clinical skill level: 3

❏ Following cardiac surgery the nurse constantly monitors adequate tissue perfusion. A cardinal sign of arterial obstruction is:
   1. Falling blood pressure
   2. Cardiac tamponade
   3. Decreasing cardiac output
   4. Absence of any pulse

   Answer: 4. Absence of any pulse
   Rationale: If any pulse is absent in any extremity, the physician should be notified immediately.
   Nursing process: Assessment
   Client need: Physiological integrity

   Clinical skill level: 3

❑ While monitoring cardiac output following cardiac surgery, the nurse knows the most common cause of decreasing CO is:
1. Hypovolemia
2. Hypervolemia
3. Hypokalemia
4. Hypocalcemia

Answer: 1. Hypovolemia

Rationale: Inherent in this procedure are several causes of hypovolemia:
1. Blood loss during surgery
2. Persistent bleeding following surgery
3. Loss of IV fluids into interstitial spaces due to increased permeability in the capillary beds
4. Administration of heparin

Nursing process: Assessment

Client need: Physiological integrity

Clinical skill level: 3

■ Post-cardiac surgery the nurse assesses the patient is becoming restless, confused, and weak. Hyperkalemia is suggested. Which ECG change is most likely to occur:
1. Flat, inverted T waves
2. Tall, peaked T waves
3. Third degree AV block
4. Short QT interval

Answer: 2. Tall, peaked T waves

Rationale: ECG changes specific to hyperkalemia are peaked T waves, widening QRS complex, and a prolonged QT interval.

Nursing process: Assessment

Client need: Physiological integrity

Clinical skill level: 4

❏ The nurse closely monitors the ECG on the cardiac patient post-surgery. A specific change is noted: a U wave almost 1 1/2 mm high. This is a significant sign of:
1. Hyperkalemia
2. Hypokalemia
3. Hypernatremia
4. Hyponatremia

Answer: 2. Hypokalemia

Rationale: The stress of cardiac surgery produces increased aldosterone secretion, which in turn causes decreased potassium and increased sodium.

Nursing process: Evaluation

Client need: Physiological integrity

Clinical skill level: 4

❏ The nurse reports to the physician a flat T wave on the ECG of a cardiac patient post-surgery. The nurse prepares to administer:
1. Normal saline
2. Lactated Ringer's
3. Sodium bicarbonate
4. Potassium replacement

Answer: 4. Potassium replacement

Rationale: Normal serum potassium levels must be maintained (3.5-5.0 m Eg/L) to avoid dysrhythmias postoperatively.

Nursing process: Intervention

Client need: Physiological integrity

Clinical skill level: 3

❏ A post-op assessment of the cardiac surgery patient reveals cool moist skin, dusky tone, and cyanosis in the buccal mucosa and nail beds. The nurse suspects:
1. High CVP
2. Decreasing cardiac output
3. Myocardial infarction
4. Fatal dysrhythmias

Answer: 2. Decreasing cardiac output
Rationale: These signs are all indicative of vasoconstriction and decreased cardiac output.
Nursing process: Assessment
Client need: Physiological integrity

Clinical skill level: 3

❏ During auscultation of breath sounds, the nurse notes fine crackles. This is indicative of:
1. Bacterial pneumonia
2. Cardiac dysrhythmias
3. Congestive heart failure
4. Pulmonary congestion

Answer: 4. Pulmonary congestion
Rationale: One of the first signs of fluid in the lungs is adventitious breath sounds.
Nursing process: Assessment
Client need: Physiological integrity

Clinical skill level: 2

❏ When performing an assessment, the nurse asks the patient to touch one of his fingers, his nose, then repeat the process at least three times. What is being determined by this assessment?
1. Accommodation
2. PEARLA
3. Coordination
4. Dexterity

Answer: 3. Coordination

Rationale: This coordination test is a basic neurological assessment.

Nursing process: Assessment

Client need: Physiological integrity

Clinical skill level: 1

❏ Morphine sulfate is classified as a:
1. Synthetic narcotic
2. Non-narcotic analgesic
3. Narcotic analgesic
4. Narcotic antagonist

Answer: 3. Narcotic analgesic

Rationale: Morphine is a derivative of opium and a widely-used analgesic and sedative.

Nursing process: Evaluation

Client need: Physiological integrity

Clinical skill level: 2

❏ The physician has prescribed morphine sulfate. The drug is controlled under:
1. Schedule I
2. Schedule II
3. Schedule III
4. Schedule IV

Answer: 2. Schedule II
Rationale: Morphine is a narcotic that is strictly controlled.
Nursing process: Evaluation
Client need: Physiological integrity

Clinical skill level: 2

❏ Before administering a narcotic, the nurse must:
1. Take the patient's temperature
2. Count the patient's respiratory rate
3. Be sure the patient is in enough pain
4. Have patient cough and deep breathe

Answer: 2. Count the patient's respiratory rate
Rationale: Narcotics tend to depres the CNS and particularly the respiratory rate. Therefore, the rate must be within normal limits. This reading also serves as a baseline for evaluating the effects of the medication.
Nursing process: Outcome criteria
Client need: Physiological integrity

Clinical skill level: 2

❏ In addition to respiratory rate, which important assessment should the nurse document approximately 15-30 minutes after administering a narcotic?
1. Temperature
2. Response
3. Hypertension
4. Constipation

Answer: 2. Response

Rationale: The nurse should evaluate the response to medication to assess if patient is getting adequate pain relief. If not, the physician should be notified.

Nursing process: Outcome criteria

Client need: Physiological integrity

Clinical skill level: 2

❏ When administering Heparin, the nurse should remember:
1. To massage injection site
2. Do not massage injection site
3. To give deep IM with 18 gauge needle
4. To give IV push only

Answer: 2. Do not massage injection site

Rationale: Heparin is an anticoagulant that should be injected at rotated sites around the stomach. Massage, or aspiration, may cause the formation of a hematoma.

Nursing process: Intervention

Client need: Physiological integrity

Clinical skill level: 2

❑ In assessing a patient with insomnia, the nurse is aware that the most common cause of sleeplessness is:
1. Drug abuse
2. Jet lag
3. Depression
4. Poor sleep habits

Answer: 4. Poor sleep habits

Rationale: When a patient suffers insomnia, the nurse should assess and encourage habits such as regular bedtime, nutritional intake and bedtime rituals.

Nursing process: Assessment

Client need: Health promotion and maintenance

Clinical skill level: 2

❑ What is the legal aspect with which nurses would be held liable when giving emergency care?
1. Complications arising from injuries
2. Injury resulting from mistakes made accidentally
3. Not stopping at scene of accident
4. Temporarily functioning in the physician role

Answer: 4. Temporarily functioning in the physician role

Rationale: Usually nurses are protected by Good Samaritan laws in an emergency outside the hospital. However, these laws will cover the nurse only as long as she performs duties that are legal under the Nurse Practice Act in the state in which she is licensed. She cannot perform the duties of a physician.

Nursing process: Assessment

Client need: Health promotion and maintenance

Clinical skill level: 2

❏ Under the Good Samaritan law, when can a nurse be charged with abandonment in an emergency situation?
   1. If she doesn't stop and render aid
   2. If she begins aid and abruptly stops
   3. If she does not initiate appropriate trauma care
   4. If she does not act under a physician's orders

   Answer: 2. If she begins aid and abruptly stops

   Rationale: Once aid is initiated, the nurse is responsible for doing everything she can under the circumstances for the good of the patient. If she interrupts care, she may be charged with abandonment.

   Nursing process: Intervention

   Client need: Health promotion and maintenance

   Clinical skill level: 2

4. Nurses may be judged negligent when they:
   1. Violate standards of care
   2. Act in good faith but make mistakes
   3. Make a medication error that does not harm the patient
   4. Delegate appropriate duties to other staff members

   Answer: 1. Violate standards of care

   Rationale: The nurse is professionally obligated to the standards of care dictated by the profession, depending upon the education or experience she possesses.

   Nursing process: Intervention

   Client need: Physiological integrity

   Clinical skill level: 2

❏ Which of the following legal concepts is most important for the nurse to develop?
1. Assertiveness
2. Dedication
3. Humility
4. Accountability

Answer: 4. Accountability

Rationale: The practice of professional nursing is based on the concept of accountability. This means that the nurse is responsible for her actions and can be held accountable for those actions.

Nursing process: Intervention

Client need: Safe, effective care environment

Clinical skill level: 1

❏ The nurse is told by the physician he suspects meningitis in a 26-year-old female patient who is admitted with 106 degree fever. In assessing for this condition, the nurse performs a:
1. Homan's sign
2. Kernig's sign
3. Chadwick's sign
4. Brudinski's sign

Answer: 2. Kernig's sign

Rationale: Kernig's sign is positive if the patient complains of pain in the back or back of the leg when the leg is raised while the hip and knee are flexed. A positive Kernig's sign is part of the diagnostic criteria for meningitis.

Nursing process: Evaluation

Client need: Physiological integrity

Clinical skill level: 2

❏ Where is peripheral cyanosis first assessed?
1. Eyes
2. Tip of nose
3. Nailbeds
4. Tongue

Answer: 2. Tip of nose

Rationale: Peripheral vasoconstriction causes cyanosis in the nailbeds before spreading throughout the body.

Nursing process: Assessment

Client need: Physiological integrity

Clinical skill level: 2

❏ Heparin is available in a 2 ml vial, 20,000 units per ml. The order reads 20,000 units in 500 ml D5W at 1000 units/hr. The nurse will set the infusion pump at:
1. 10 ml/hr.
2. 20 ml/hr.
3. 25 ml/hr.
4. 50 ml/hr.

Answer: 3. 25 ml/hr.

Rationale: 20,000 units in 500 ml = 40 units/ml. 1000 ml/hr. = 40 units/ml. = 25 ml.hr

Nursing process: Intervention

Client need: Physiological integrity

Clinical skill level: 2

❏ Research indicates the most important component in handwashing, other than soap and water, is:
1. Betadine
2. Dry towel
3. Friction
4. Lotion

Answer: 3. Friction

Rationale: Friction has been cited as almost as important as soap in adequate handwashing techniques.

Nursing process: Intervention

Client need: Physiological integrity

Clinical skill level: 1

❏ A positive Homan's sign is found in a post-op patient. An immediate priority is:
1. Strict bedrest
2. IV antibiotics
3. Early ambulation
4. Pain medication

Answer: 1. Strict bedrest

Rationale: A positive Homan's sign is indicative of thrombophlebitis, a serious complication following surgery. The patient should be immobilized with affected leg elevated.

Nursing process: Intervention

Client need: Physiological integrity

Clinical skill level: 3

❏ Anticonvulsant therapy is initiated for a patient who is experiencing seizures. The nurse instructs that the medication should be taken:
1. In the morning
2. Between meals
3. With meals only
4. At bedtime

Answer: 4. At bedtime

Rationale: Anticonvulsants cause drowsiness, and this side effect decreases with the h.s. administration.

Nursing process: Intervention

Client need: Physiological integrity

Clinical skill level: 2

❏ The nurse is performing an initial assessment on a 58-year-old man complaining of pain in his left leg. He also describes numbness and tingling. The nurse suspects a circulatory problem. Her most important physical assessment is:
1. Checking the carotid pulse
2. Checking the popliteal pulse
3. Blood pressure and capillary refill
4. Assessing a limp in the left leg

Answer: 2. Checking the popliteal pulse

Rationale: The popliteal pulse is the best indicator of circulation in the legs.

Nursing process: Assessment

Client need: Physiological integrity

Clinical skill level: 2

❏ The nurse teaches that the best exercise for a patient with peripheral vascular disease is:
   1. Leg lifts
   2. Jogging
   3. Walking
   4. Rotation leg exercises

   Answer: 3. Walking

   Rationale: Walking is the best way to improve impaired collateral circulation.

   Nursing process: Intervention

   Client need: Physiological integrity

   Clinical skill level: 3

❏ The nurse assesses a jagged cut on a patient injured in a car accident. Tearing of the skin's surface is called a/an:
   1. Wheal
   2. Fissure
   3. Abrasion
   4. Laceration

   Answer: 4. Laceration

   Rationale: A laceration occurs when the skin is torn roughly, and the edges are uneven.

   Nursing process: Assessment

   Client need: Physiological integrity

   Clinical skill level: 1

❏ Dreams are more vivid during which stage of sleep?
   1. REM
   2. NonREM stage II
   3. NonREM stage III
   4. NonREM stage IV

   Answer: 1. REM

   Rationale: REM sleep begins about 90 minutes after a person falls asleep. It is the second stage of sleep and is characterized by quick eye movement and dreaming.

   Nursing process: Outcome criteria

   Client need: Health promotion and maintenance

   Clinical skill level: 2

❏ The familiar biorhythm is the day/night cycle known as the:
   1. Circadian rhythm
   2. Biological rhythm
   3. REM rhythm
   4. Psychological rhythm

   Answer: 1. Circadian rhythm

   Rationale: The Circadian rhythm consists of sleeping and waking patterns that occur in a 24-hour period. The rhythm tends to repeat itself automatically. It determines a person's high and low periods of cognitive functioning.

   Nursing process: Assessment

   Client need: Health promotion and maintenance

   Clinical skill level: 2

❑ Sleep is believed to be produced by the release of:
   1. Epinephrine
   2. Endorphins
   3. Serotonin
   4. Acetacholine

   Answer: 3. Serotonin

   Rationale: Serotonin is a hormone mediator which synthesizes a hypnogenic factor that directly causes sleep.

   Nursing process: Assessment
   Client need: Physiological integrity

   Clinical skill level: 2

❑ Decubitus ulcers result primarily from:
   1. Prolonged illness
   2. Restricted mobility
   3. Pressure on bony prominences
   4. Sloughing of the skin

   Answer: 3. Pressure on bony prominences

   Rationale: Immobility and inactivity contribute to the occurrence of decubitus, due to prolonged periods of pressure on bony prominences, and diminished circulation to the tissues.

   Nursing process: Assessment
   Client need: Health promotion and maintenance

   Clinical skill level: 1

❏ When assessing skin of an immobilized patient, the nurse should carefully note:
1. Color and moisture of the mucous membranes
2. Distribution and texture of body hair
3. Skin turgor and bony prominences
4. Distribution of body fat

Answer: 3. Skin turgor and bony prominences

Rationale: An immobilized patient will have the greatest difficulty preventing pressure ulcers created by shearing forces and friction. Therefore, the skin should first be assessed for characteristics that would predispose to decubitus formation.

Nursing process: Assessment

Client need: Physiological integrity

Clinical skill level: 1

❏ Embolic stockings are prescribed for the immobilized patient primarily because they:
1. Promote ROM
2. Impede venous return
3. Promote venous return
4. Prevent contractors

Answer: 3. Promote venous return

Rationale: The slight pressure of the support stockings reduces pooling of blood in the legs and increases blood return to the heart.

Nursing process: Outcome criteria

Client need: Health promotion and maintenance

Clinical skill level: 1

❏ When assessing an immobilized patient for edema, the area to check initially is:
1. Face and neck
2. Feet and legs
3. Arms and hands
4. Abdomen

Answer: 2. Feet and legs

Rationale: When circulation is impaired, fluid is first pooled in the extremities.

Nursing process: Assessment

Client need: Physiological integrity

Clinical skill level: 2

❏ The sleep cycle in which it is difficult to arouse the patient and which is believed responsible for restoring and healing the body is:
1. NonREM stage II
2. NonREM stage III
3. NonREM stage IV
4. REM sleep

Answer: 3. NonREM stage IV

Rationale: The EEG reveals that stage IV is a deep, slow-wave sleep. Non-REM sleep is predominant at the beginning of the sleep cycle and REM is more predominant at the end. Both REM and non-REM sleep are essential for physiologic and psychologic integrity.

Nursing process: Assessment

Client need: Physiological/psychological integrity

Clinical skill level: 2

❏ An intervention that would encourage sleep and focus on the patient goal of obtaining a sense of restfulness is:
1. Encouraging ambulation for 10 minutes one hour before bedtime
2. Providing the patient with a cookie, hot tea, and lemon one hour before bedtime
3. Having patient sit in a chair for two hours before retiring
4. Suggesting the patient read a novel or watch TV before retiring

Answer: 2. Providing the patient with a cookie, hot tea, and lemon before bedtime

Rationale: Research shows that simple glucose and a warm liquid promotes the secretion of serotonin, which promotes sleep.

Nursing process: Intervention

Client need: Health promotion and maintenance

Clinical skill level: 2

❏ The patient with athlete's foot is taught to:
1. Avoid walking barefoot
2. Wash feet after swimming
3. Soak feet in warm salt water
4. Keep feet dry and go barefoot when possible

Answer: 4. Keep feet dry and go barefoot when possible

Rationale: Keeping the feet dry prevents new growth of fungi; the dryness and air also promotes healing as fungi prefer dark, moist environments.

Nursing process: Intervention

Client need: Health promotion and maintenance

Clinical skill level: 2

❏ To reduce the neuralgia for an older person with herpes zoster, the physician may prescribe:
1. Anti-fungal topicals
2. Systemic anti-fungals
3. Systemic antibiotics
4. Systemic corticosteroids

Answer: 4. Systemic corticosteroids

Rationale: Systemic corticosteroids reduce inflammation and shorten the course of herpes. Steroids do not have anti-viral properties.

Nursing process: Outcome criteria

Client need: Physiological integrity

Clinical skill level: 2

❏ Herpes zoster, or shingles, is characterized by clusters of vesicles that follow the pathway of sensory nerves on the back, face, and scalp. The major problem with herpes zoster is:
1. Resistance to antibiotics
2. Pain and itching
3. Difficult to heal
4. No effective therapy

Answer: 2. Pain and itching

Rationale: Because herpes zoster follows the nerve pathway, it is especially painful.

Nursing process: Outcome criteria

Client need: Physiological integrity

Clinical skill level: 2

❑ A patient has been diagnosed with a bacterial infection, cellulitis, in the left leg. The physician prescribes systemic antibiotics, elevation of the leg, and rest. In planning care, the nurse knows rest is of utmost importance because rest:
1. Keeps body temperature down
2. Aids work of antibiotics
3. Prevents spread of infection
4. Aids in decreasing fever

Answer: 3. Prevents spread of infection

Rationale: Activity causes muscle contractions that could introduce the bacterial organism into the blood stream and spread into the surrounding tissue.

Nursing process: Outcome criteria

Client need: Physiological integrity

Clinical skill level: 2

❑ A patient is brought into the ER with a narcotic overdose. The nurse prepares to administer:
1. Lasix IV
2. Narcan IV
3. Solu-medrol
4. Epinephrine

Answer: 2. Narcan IV

Rationale: Narcan is a narcotic antagonist which quickly reverses their CNS depressant effects.

Nursing process: Intervention

Client need: Physiological integrity

Clinical skill level: 3

❏ Dopamine is administered to maintain:
1. Potassium levels
2. Digestive functioning
3. And stimulate urinary output
4. And stimulate perfusion to organs

Answer: 4. And stimulate perfusion to organs

Rationale: Dopamine stimulates receptors of the sympathetic nervous system and is used to treat shock, hypotension, and to increase cardiac output.

Nursing process: Intervention

Client need: Physiological integrity

| Clinical skill level: 3 |

❏ What is the first priority in the assessment of an injured person?
1. Fractures
2. Level of consciousness
3. Hemorrhage
4. Airway status

Answer: 4. Airway status

Rationale: Although the other injuries may be critical, airway status is always the priority in any assessment.

Nursing process: Assessment

Client need: Physiological integrity

| Clinical skill level: 2 |

❏ In a head-to-toe assessment under emergency conditions, what is checked first?
1. Pupils
2. Carotids
3. Airway
4. Cervical spine

Answer: 3. Airway

Rationale: If the airway is blocked, the priority intervention will be directed toward initiating breathing, whether spontaneously or mechanically.

Nursing process: Assessment

Client need: Physiological integrity

Clinical skill level: 2

❏ A person who has just swallowed a poisonous mushroom should be given:
1. 15 ml of syrup of Ipecac and water
2. Milk in copious amounts with water
3. One glass of water with teaspoon of salt
4. Teaspoon of bicarbonate soda with water

Answer: 1. 15 ml of syrup of Ipecac and water

Rationale: The treatment for mushroom poisoning is similar to treatment for drug poisoning: induce vomiting with Ipecac and flush body with fluids.

Nursing process: Intervention

Client need: Physiological integrity

Clinical skill level: 3

❏ Intensive care unit patients who are NPO are at high risk for stress ulcers. The medication that is prescribed to inhibit this complication is:
1. Tagamet
2. Valium
3. Pavulon
4. Morphine

Answer: 1. Tagamet

Rationale: Tagamet (cimetidine) decreases the secretion of gastric acid by inhibiting the action of histamine.

Nursing process: Intervention

Client need: Physiological integrity

Clinical skill level: 3

❏ In a trauma center, one of the nurse's responsibility is to triage. What specific action is involved?
1. Managing patients critically injured in a disaster
2. Initiating primary care in absence of a physician
3. Ordering initial lab work, x-rays, starting an IV
4. Sorting patients according to priority of care for their condition

Answer: 4. Sorting patients according to priority of care for their condition

Rationale: The triage nurse must decide the priority in which any patient who comes to the ER will require emergency care and make most efficient use of medical and nursing services.

Nursing process: Assessment

Client need: Physiological integrity

Clinical skill level: 2

❏ The patient in the emergency room asks for a drink of water. The nurse checks the chart and finds his chief complaint is abdominal pain. The priority is to:
1. Give him water
2. Withhold fluids
3. Give him juice
4. Check with doctor

Answer: 2. Withhold fluids

Rationale: This patient may require surgery and should be held NPO until the physician makes a determination. Fluids or foods could cause pneumonia if aspirated.

Nursing process: Intervention

Client need: Physiological integrity

Clinical skill level: 3

❏ A patient is in the recovery room following intermaxillary fixation for a fractured jaw. Two hours after surgery he begins to vomit. The nurse should:
1. Cut the wires so the vomitus can be expelled
2. Position in High Fowler's with head forward
3. Call the physician to insert an endotracheal tube
4. Administer an antiemetic IM as ordered

Answer: 1. Cut the wires so the vomitus can be expelled

Rationale: If the wires are not cut immediately, the vomitus could be aspirated, perhaps causing a respiratory emergency.

Nursing process: Intervention

Client need: Physiological integrity

Clinical skill level: 3

❏ The patient with tic douloureux should be carefully assessed for undernourishment and dehydration because:
1. Chewing is exceedingly painful
2. Nutrients are easily depleted
3. Swallowing is very difficult
4. Vomiting is a frequent problem

Answer: 1. Chewing is exceedingly painful

Rationale: Trigeminal neuralgia, a painful condition of cranial nerve V causes dysfunction in chewing.

Nursing process: Evaluation

Client need: Physiological integrity

Clinical skill level: 3

❏ The drug of choice in treating tic douloureux is:
1. Stadol
2. Demerol
3. Tegretol
4. Morphine

Answer: 3. Tegretol

Rationale: Carbamazepine (Tegretol) relieves the pain by partially inhibiting the transmission nerve impulses. Phenytoin (Dilantin) also may be prescribed.

Nursing process: Intervention

Client need: Physiological integrity

Clinical skill level: 3

❑ In assessing a patient with trigeminal neuralgia, or tic douloureux, the nurse knows it is characterized by:
1. Blindness
2. Paralysis
3. Tremors
4. Intense pain

Answer: 4. Intense pain

Rationale: One of the clinical manifestations of a disorder of cranial nerve V, the trigeminal nerve, is facial pain. Patients describe it as an electrical shock or an intense burning sensation.

Nursing process: Assessment

Client need: Physiological integrity

> Clinical skill level: 2

■ The nurse assesses a cancer patient who is receiving chemotherapy and has developed diffuse petechiae. The lab results reveal very low RBCs. What side effect of chemotherapy accounts for this assessment data?
1. Low white blood count
2. Increased lymphocytes
3. Diminished platelets
4. Bone marrow suppression

Answer: 3. Diminished platelets

Rationale: Petechiae occutrs most commonly in platelet disorders and is one of the first signs of decreasing platelets and capillary fragility.

Nursing process: Evaluation

Client need: Physiological integrity

> Clinical skill level: 4

❏ The drug that acts as an antagonist for Coumadin is:
1. Vitamin A
2. Vitamin E
3. Vitamin K
4. Protamine sulfate

Answer: 3. Vitamin K

Rationale: Because Coumadin inhibits the synthesis of Vitamin K, injections may be required to decrease the risk of bleeding. The effects of Vitamin K are not immediate, however. It may take 10-14 days for Vitamin K to take effect.

Nursing process: Intervention

Client need: Physiological integrity

Clinical skill level: 3

❏ The patient on Lasix complains of muscle cramps, apathy and general malaise. The nurse suspects:
1. Sodium depletion
2. Potassium depletion
3. Noncompliance with medication
4. Generalized depression

Answer: 2. Potassium depletion

Rationale: The symptoms listed are indications of hypokalemia.

Nursing process: Evaluation

Client need: Physiological integrity

Clinical skill level: 3

❏ The patient is extremely hypoxic. Which assessment indicates the body is attempting to compensate?
1. Decreased urinary output
2. Decreasing blood pressure
3. Increasing blood pressure
4. Increased respirations and heart rate

Answer: 4. Increased respirations and heart rate

Rationale: The body will attempt to pump more blood to oxygenate the body, and respirations will increase in order to blow off CO_2.

Nursing process: Outcome criteria

Client need: Physiological integrity

Clinical skill level: 3

❏ The catecholamines, epinephrine and norepinephrine, have different effects on the body. Basically, they:
1. Maintain feedback system
2. Maintain homeostasis
3. Control heart rate
4. Control hormones

Answer: 2. Maintain homeostasis

Rationale: These hormones constrict blood vessels, however, they are selective in their actions. Epinephrine acts in small doses to offset norepinephrine by dilating vessels to the muscles, brain, and heart.

Nursing process: Evaluation

Client need: Physiological integrity

Clinical skill level: 2

❑ The result of a prothrombin time is 25 sec. This indicates a prolonged clotting time. What does this mean to the nurse?
   1. No special precautions are necessary
   2. Spontaneous bleeding could occur
   3. Liver functioning is impaired
   4. Blood transfusion may be necessary

   Answer: 2. Spontaneous bleeding could occur
   Rationale: The normal PT is 9-12 seconds. A PT of twice that indicates the patient is at risk for a bleeding disorder.
   Nursing process: Assessment
   Client need: Physiological integrity

   Clinical skill level: 2

❑ The patient asks the nurse to explain the etiology of migraine headaches. The nurse answers based on pathophysiology that is characteristic of migraines:
   1. Vessels constrict, restricting blood flow
   2. Vessels become clogged, reducing blood flow
   3. Vessels dilate, becoming congested
   4. Vessels dilate, emptying vessels too quickly

   Answer: 1. Vessels constrict, restricting blood flow
   Rationale: The vascular theory states that migraines are caused by constriction of vessels, therefore blood flow throughout the brain is reduced during a migraine.
   Nursing process: Intervention
   Client need: Physiological integrity

   Clinical skill level: 2

❏ The nursing assessment is: flexion of arms, wrists, fingers, adduction of upper extremities. The nurse documents this condition as:
1. Cerebrovascular accident
2. Epileptic seizure
3. Decorticate posturing
4. Decerebrate posturing

Answer: 3. Decorticate posturing

Rationale: The patient who has suffered injury to the central nervous system may exhibit decorticate posturing.

Nursing process: Assessment

Client need: Physiological integrity

Clinical skill level: 2

❏ Decorticate posturing is the result of:
1. Loss of consciousness
2. Injury to the brain stem
3. Loss of motor functioning
4. Loss of sensorimotor function

Answer: 2. Injury to brain stem

Rationale: Decorticate posturing is the abnormal manifestation of impingement on the motor pathways of the brainstem.

Nursing process: Assessment

Client need: Physiological integrity

Clinical skill level: 2

❏   A score of five on the Glasgow Coma Scale is assessed. This assessment indicates that the patient is:
   1. Alert and oriented
   2. In shock
   3. Responding appropriately
   4. Not responsive

   Answer: 4. Not responsive

   Rationale: When assessing a patient according to the Glasgow Coma Scale, 15 is the highest score in which a patient is still alert and oriented. The lower the score, the less responsive the patient.

   Nursing process: Evaluation

   Client need: Physiological integrity

   Clinical skill level: 2

❏   Patient education for the person with psoriasis includes:
   1. Modifying lifestyle
   2. Managing stress
   3. Avoiding sunlight
   4. Coping with pain

   Answer: 2. Managing stress

   Rationale: Psoriasis is believed to be exacerbated by stress. There is no cure for psoriasis, but tends to improve with healthy lifestyle and exposure to UV light.

   Nursing process: Outcome criteria

   Client need: Physiological integrity

   Clinical skill level: 2

❑ To prevent post-operative pulmonary complications, pre-operatively, the nurse will intervene by:
1. Asking the doctor to order IPPB
2. Teaching stomach and leg exercises
3. Teaching use of a flow-oriented incentive spirometer
4. Telling him that if he does not cough, he will be suctioned

Answer: 3. Teaching use of a flow-oriented incentive spirometer

Rationale: Incentive spirometry encourages diaphragmatic breathing necessary to keep airways clear.

Nursing process: Intervention

Client need: Physiological integrity

> Clinical skill level: 2

❑ The nurse is monitoring a paraplegic patient. A common complication the nurse should be alert to is:
1. Bradycardia
2. High blood pressure
3. Slow capillary refill
4. Postural hypotension

Answer: 4. Postural hypotension

Rationale: In paraplegics, the vasoconstriction that normally occurs upon arising has been interrupted, and pooling of venous blood causes decreased blood flow to the heart, resulting in hypotension.

Nursing process: Assessment

Client need: Physiological integrity

> Clinical skill level: 2

❑ A decrease of calcium in the body causes:
1. Anemia
2. Weakness
3. Seizures
4. Tetany

Answer: 4. Tetany

Rationale: Increased neuromuscular irritability as manifested by, tingling in extremities, positive Chvostek's sign and positive Trousseau's sign are indicative of low calcium levels.

Nursing process: Assessment

Client need: Physiological integrity

Clinical skill level: 2

❑ When planning for a patient in restraints, the care plan should emphasize that restraints should be removed:
1. Every hour
2. Every 2 hours
3. Every 4 hours
4. Every 8 hours

Answer: 3. Every 4 hours

Rationale: Restraints should be removed regularly to allow the patient to move freely and to promote circulation.

Nursing process: Intervention

Client need: Physiological integrity

Clinical skill level: 2

❑ After removing restraints, what safety measure must be implemented?
1. Document patient response
2. Let down side rails
3. Do not leave patient unattended
4. Attach restraints to side rail

Answer: 3. Do not leave patient unattended

Rationale: It would be unsafe to leave the patient unrestrained and unattended.

Nursing process: Intervention

Client need: Physiological integrity

Clinical skill level: 3

❑ The nurse is assisting in a thoracentesis. She is aware that the needle will be inserted into the:
1. Lungs
2. Thorax
3. Pleural space
4. Bronchi

Answer: 3. Pleural space

Rationale: One of the purposes of the thoracentesis is to remove air or fluid from the pleural space. The procedure is also sometimes performed for diagnostic purposes.

Nursing process: Outcome criteria

Client need: Physiological integrity

Clinical skill level: 2

❑ In assessing a patient has a potential fluid-electrolyte imbalance, the nurse is aware that the largest amount of body fluids is found in which compartment?
1. Extracellular
2. Interstitial
3. Transcellular
4. Intracellular

Answer: 4. Intracellular

Rationale: Intracellular fluid is within the cells and is instrumental in the chemical functions of the cell. About two-thirds of the body's fluid is intracellular and one-third is extracellular.

Nursing process: Assessment

Client need: Physiological integrity

Clinical skill level: 2

❑ A trauma patient has a clear fluid draining from his nose. How will the nurse determine if the drainage is spinal fluid?
1. Perform a spinal tap
2. Use a Dextrostix to identify glucose
3. Test the drainage for the presence of bacteria
4. Order a blood sugar

Answer: 2. Use a Dextrostix to identify glucose

Rationale: Spinal fluid contains glucose. A quick way to assess if glucose is present is to test it with a dextrostix.

Nursing process: Assessment

Client need: Physiological integrity

Clinical skill level: 3

❏ The patient is scheduled for thoracentesis. Which information is included in the teaching plan?
1. Explain that the procedure will not hurt
2. Caution that he must not move or cough for 6 hours post-procedure
3. Explain that he will be positioned sitting on the edge of the bed with arms and head on the bedside table
4. Explain to him that the needle will be left in place to drain

Answer: 3. Explain that he will be positioned sitting on the edge of the bed with arms and head on the bedside table

Rationale: This position is optimal for expansion of the chest wall. This position facilitates the insertion of the needle.

Nursing process: Intervention

Client need: Physiological integrity

Clinical skill level: 2

❏ Alice Jones, RN, is circulating in the operating room. She accidentally brushes her arm against the front of your gown. You are the scrub nurse today. The priority action is:
1. Ignore it because she is also sterile
2. To avoid disruption and creating hard feelings, ignore it
3. Tell her it is her job to be more careful
4. Request a new gown; contamination has occurred

Answer: 4. Request a new gown; contamination has occurred

Rationale: The circulatory nurse is a nonsterile member of the OR team. Any contact will contaminate a sterile member.

Nursing process: Intervention

Client need: Physiological integrity

Clinical skill level: 2

❏ In transferring a post-operative patient, the main concern is to avoid:
1. Strain on the incision
2. Breaking the IV bottles
3. Dislodging a blood clot
4. Increasing the patient's pain

Answer: 1. Strain on the incision

Rationale: Strain on a new incision may cause hemorrhage or other complications such as evisceration.

Nursing process: Intervention

Client need: Physiological integrity

Clinical skill level: 2

❏ The patient is in the recovery room after a long surgery. He is unconscious and is lying on his back. The nurse observes that his respirations are irregular and noisy. He begins choking and is cyanotic. The priority nursing intervention is:
1. Call the physician
2. Raise the head of the bed
3. Administer oxygen
4. Tilt the head back and push forward on the angle of the lower jaw

Answer: 4. Tilt the head back and push forward on the angle of the lower jaw

Rationale: This patient may be suffering an airway obstruction. This movement is best to open airway and remove obstruction.

Nursing process: Intervention

Client need: Physiological integrity

Clinical skill level: 3

❏ A 68-year-old patient suddenly refuses to sign the operative permit for amputation of his left leg. The nurse contacts the physician. The expected action is to:
1. Declare the patient mentally incompetent
2. Ask the daughter to sign the permit
3. Cancel the surgery
4. Give an ultimatum to the patient

Answer: 3. Cancel the surgery

Rationale: The surgeon most likely will not initiate the surgery without a signed informed consent.

Nursing process: Intervention

Client need: Physiological integrity

Clinical skill level: 2

❏ Pre-operative teaching in the areas of turning, coughing, deep breathing, range of motion exercises, and splinting the wound. Which of the following would also have been most appropriate was done with a patient scheduled for abdominal surgery?
1. Pain control post-operatively
2. How to manage at home post-operatively
3. Advise on how to cope with hemorrhage
4. Anticipatory guidance regarding diet post-operatively

Answer: 1. Pain control post-operatively

Rationale: Research indicates that patients respond more positively when they know pain medication is available and when they have some control in the administration of medication.

Nursing process: Intervention

Client need: Physiological integrity

Clinical skill level: 3

☐ The patient is quite unhappy about having food withheld prior to abdominal surgery. The nurse explains that the reason is to:
1. Keep the stomach size reduced
2. Decrease intestinal activity and pulmonary complications
3. Prevent aspiration and pulmonary complications
4. Cleanse the GI tract and reduce bacteria

Answer: 3. Prevent aspiration and pulmonary complications

Rationale: Anesthesia may cause the patient to vomit and aspirate the contents into the lungs, causing dangerous respiratory complications.

Nursing process: Intervention

Client need: Physiological integrity

Clinical skill level: 2

☐ The nurse is preparing to administer the pre-op medication to a patient scheduled for surgery. One of the last things the nurse should do in completing the pre-operative checklist is:
1. Have the priest say a prayer
2. Have the client void
3. Ask the patient if he needs a drink
4. Have the patient sign the operative permit

Answer: 2. Have the client void

Rationale: The anxiety of surgery may cause the patient to urinate more frequently than usual, and the patient should be prepared for transport when the team arrives.

Nursing process: Intervention

Client need: Physiological integrity

Clinical skill level: 2

❏ Atropine was administered as a pre-anesthetic medication. Atropine is:
1. An anticholinergic used to reduce respiratory tract secretions
2. An opiate used to reduce amount of anesthesia required
3. A barbiturate used to produce sedation prior to surgery
4. An antibiotic used prophylactically to reduce infection

Answer: 1. An anti-cholinergic used to reduce respiratory tract secretions

Rationale Atropine dries the secretions that are produced when the vagal nerve is stimulated during surgery.

Nursing process: Intervention

Client need: Physiological integrity

Clinical skill level: 2

❏ Tylenol has few side effects. However, one of the important complications that too much Tylenol can cause is:
1. Kidney damage
2. Liver damage
3. Decrease in WBC count
4. Decrease in spleen production

Answer: 2. Liver damage

Rationale: Tylenol is metabolized by the liver and is highly toxic in large amounts.

Nursing process: Evaluation

Client need: Physiological integrity

Clinical skill level: 2

❏ Which complication of wound healing is a medical emergency?
1. Drainage
2. Infection
3. Fistula
4. Evisceration

Answer: 4. Evisceration

Rationale: Evisceration occurs when internal organs protrude from the wound.

Nursing process: Assessment

Client need: Physiological integrity

Clinical skill level: 2

❏ A patient is diagnosed with a ruptured appendix. If left untreated this will cause:
1. Hypovolemic shock
2. Peritonitis
3. Hypertensive crisis
4. Meckel's diverticulum

Answer: 2. Peritonitis

Rationale: When the appendix ruptures, contaminated fluids drain into the peritoneal cavity and become a source of infection.

Nursing process: Assessment

Client need: Physiological integrity

Clinical skill level: 2

❏ Which of the following best states the rationale for assessing pre-operative vital signs?
  1. Complies with standard policy on all client admitted to the hospital
  2. Helps determine which anesthetic should be given
  3. Provides a baseline to assist in determining pre-existing problems
  4. Reassures the patient that he is being cared for appropriately

  Answer: 3. Provides a baseline to assist in determining pre-existing problems
  Rationale: In order to evaluate vital signs in each successive reading, a baseline reading is required.
  Nursing process: Assessment
  Client need: Physiological integrity

  Clinical skill level: 2

❏ After receiving a dose of penicillin, a patient is admitted to the emergency department of a hospital with an audible expiratory wheeze, hives, and a feeling of impending doom The nurse prepares to administer:
  1. Sodium bicarbonate
  2. Epinephrine
  3. Valium IM
  4. Norepinephrine

  Answer: 2. Epinephrine
  Rationale: These are signs and symptoms of an anaphylaxis and epinephrine is the medication of choice.
  Nursing process: Intervention
  Client need: Physiological integrity

  Clinical skill level: 3

❑ In performing a neurological assessment, the nurse recognizes the INITIAL indication of increasing intracranial pressure is:
1. Changing pulse pressure
2. Bulging temporal mass
3. Change in sensorium and restlessness
4. Increasing respirations and pulse

Answer: 3. Change in sensorium and restless

Rationale: The first sign of IICP is restlessness.

Nursing process: Assessment

Client need: Physiological integrity

Clinical skill level: 3

❑ The patient is suffering unrelenting hiccups. The physician prescribes:
1. Tofranil
2. Sparine
3. Thorazine
4. Compazine

Answer: 3. Thorazine

Rationale: Thorazine is a phenothiazine that is classified as an antipsychotic and antiemetic medication. It acts to block postsynaptic dopamine receptors in the brain.

Nursing process: Intervention

Client need: Physiological integrity

Clinical skill level: 3

❏ When a patient develops a tolerance to medication, the physician will likely:
1. DC the medication
2. Increase the dose
3. Decrease the dose
4. Change to another medication

Answer: 2. Increase the dose

Rationale: When a patient experiences a tolerance to medication, this means he is no longer getting the full benefit of the medication. Therefore, more medication is required to get the same effect.

Nursing process: Evaluation

Client need: Physiological integrity

Clinical skill level: 2

❏ According to Selye, stress is:
1. Determined by the nature of the threat
2. Experienced mostly by individuals who abuse substances
3. A nonspecific body response to any demand
4. Greater in addicts than non-addicts

Answer: 3. A nonspecific body response to any demand

Rationale: Selye states the body can respond in many ways to any demand, whether negative or positive. It is the body's response, and not the stressor, that is critical.

Nursing process: Assessment

Client need: Psychosocial integrity

Clinical skill level: 3

❏ If the patient is experiencing hypocalcemia, what ECG reading would correlate with this complication?
1. Tall T waves
2. Peaked U wave
3. Prolonged P-R interval
4. Prolonged Q-T interval

Answer: 4. Prolonged Q-T interval

Rationale: The Q-T interval is normally 0.38-0.40 seconds. Hypercalcemia increases it from 0.40 to 0.50 seconds.

Nursing process: Evaluation

Client need: Physiological integrity

> Clinical skill level: 4

❏ The patient is scheduled for a bone marrow aspiration. The nursing instruction includes:
1. "There will be no pain, just some discomfort."
2. "You will be under general anesthetic."
3. "There will be a brief sharp pain."
4. "You may experience pain after the procedure."

Answer: 3. "There will be a brief sharp pain during the aspiration."

Rationale: A specially designed needle is inserted into the bone and a screw-like motion removes a sample of the marrow. When the marrow is taken, a brief discomfort is experienced by the patient.

Nursing process: Intervention

Client need: Physiological integrity

> Clinical skill level: 2

■ Which is the best nursing intervention when providing care for the patient with epistaxis?
1. Lean forward and apply warm compresses to the nose
2. Lie flat and compress the upper portion of the nose
3. Set upright and compress the outer portion of the nose
4. Cough and clear the nasal passage of any clots

Answer: 3. Set upright and compress the outer portion of the nose

Rationale: Most common epistaxis can be stopped by compression for 5-10 minutes. Ice packs are also recommended. Keeping the patient upright prevents airway obstruction.

Nursing process: Intervention

Client need: Physiological integrity

Clinical skill level: 2

Index

A

ABGs, 2, 23, 34, 67, 78, 84
Accountability, 378
Acetaminophen, 203
Acquired immune deficiency syndrome (AIDS), 92
Acromegaly, 186
Addisonian crisis, 177
ADH, 185
Adult respiratory distress syndrome (ARDS), 2
AFB, 103
Alkaline ash diet, 216
Allopurinol, 121
Alopecia, 314, 316
Alveoli, 52, 64
Alzheimer's disease, 134
Aminophylline, 15, 19
Amputation, 340
Anaphylaxis, 2, 97
Anemia
    Iron deficiency, 110
    Pernicious, 122
    Sickle cell, 126
Angina pectoris, 60
Anorexia, 43, 67
Aphasia, 141
Aqueous humor, 285
Arterial blood gases, 35
Aspirin, 322
Asthma, 13, 18
Atelectasis, 2, 21, 48
Athlete's foot, 387
Atropine, 87, 409

B

Basal cell carcinoma, 313
Benadryl, 137
Benign prostatic hyperplasia, 275
Biopsy, 251
Bivalve cast, 194
Blood pressure, 74, 76
Bouchard's nodes, 200
Breath sounds, 54, 139, 323
Bronchitis, 13
Bronchogenic carcinoma, 6
Bronchoscopy, 51, 57
Buck's extension, 207
Buck's traction, 210
Buerger-Allen, 354
BUN, 219
Burns, 304
Butterfly rash, 105, 107

C

Calcium-channel blocker, 87
Calcium gluconate, 172
Cancer, 308
    Ovarian, 263
    Prostate, 272
    Warning signs of, 310
Candida infection, 313
Carbon monoxide poisoning, 10
Cardiac failure
    Left-sided, 64
    Right-sided, 67
Cardiac output, 74
Cardiac surgery, 86
Cardiogenic shock, 77
Cardiopulmonary resuscitation, 365

Cast, 188
Cast syndrome, 191
Cataracts, 280
Catecholamines, 397
Cellulitis, 389
Cerebral edema, 145
Cerebrovascular accident (CVA), 139
Chemotherapy agents, 309, 314
Chest pain, 6, 29, 43, 60, 70, 77 - 79, 89
Chest physiotherapy, 21
Cheyne-Stokes respirations, 65
Chlorpropamide (diabinese), 169
Cholecystitis, 251
Chronic obstructive pulmonary disease (COPD), 13
Chvostek's sign, 173
Circadian rhythm, 383
Circulatory status, 381
Cirrhosis of the liver, 241
Compartment syndrome, 192
Compliance, 51
Confabulation, 135
Congestive heart failure, 70
Cornea, 295
Cough, 6, 22, 43, 83, 93
Coumadin, 32
Crackles, 24, 38, 49, 64, 372
Creatine kinase (CK), 79
Cretinism, 172
Crutches, 202, 355
Crutchfield tongs, 207
Cushingoid, 180
CVP, 69
Cyanosis, 14, 22, 26, 29, 64, 83, 318, 332

D

Death, 88
Decerebrate posturing, 139
Decorticate posturing, 139
Decorticcate posturing, 399
Decubitus ulcer, 362
Decubitus ulcers, 384
Depression, 135, 178
Dexamethasone, 50
Diabetes insipidus, 168
Diabetes mellitus, 160
Diabetic ketoacidosis, 163
Diabetic retinopathy, 162
Diffusion, 52
Digitalis, 68
Disorientation, 135
Disseminated intravascular coagulopathy (DIC), 113
Diuretics, 67, 242
Dopamine, 390
Dyspnea, 2, 14, 24, 29, 43, 48, 83, 97, 110, 126
Dysuria, 222, 269

E

Edema, 196, 244, 307
Electrolyte imbalance, 4
ELISA, 94
Embolic stockings, 385
Emphysema, 13, 26, 47
Endocrine system, 159
Endorphins, 337
Endoscopy, 237
Enema, 363
Enteric precautions, 247
Epinephrine, 98

Epistaxis, 415
Evisceration, 410

F

Fat embolism, 198
Fatigue, 14, 43, 67, 70, 93, 110, 117
Fever, 6, 22, 43, 93, 101, 105, 117, 126, 204, 220, 266 - 267, 269, 309, 318, 332
Fiberglass, 188
Foley catheter, 225
Fractured jaw, 393
Fractures, 195
    Comminuted, 195
    Complete, 195
    Compression, 195
    Depressed, 195
    Displaced, 195
    Impacted, 195
    Incomplete, 195
    Open, 195
    Simple, 195
Friction rub, 31, 54

G

Gardner-Wells tongs, 207
Gastrectomy, 256
Gastrointestinal system, 235
Glasgow coma scale, 400
Glaucoma, 285, 287
Glomerulonephritis, 232
Good Samaritan law, 377

H

Haldol, 138
Handwashing, 23
Head injury, 146, 148

Headache, 74, 93
    Migraine, 398
Heart, 16
Heart sounds, 66, 73
Hematologic system, 109
Hemodialysis, 232
Hemorrhage, 318
Heparin, 368 - 369, 375, 379
Hepatitis, 241
Hepatitis A, 245
Hepatitis B, 248
Herberden's nodes, 200
Herpes zoster, 388
Hiccups, 412
Hoarseness, 8
Homan's sign, 30, 262, 380
Hypercalcemia, 183, 353
Hyperkalemia, 230, 353, 356, 360, 370
Hypertension, 60, 74, 212
Hypocalcemia, 414
Hypokalemia, 179, 356, 359 - 361, 371
Hyponatremia, 176
Hypotension, 104, 266, 318
Hypothyroidism, 170
Hypovolemia, 370
Hypovolemic shock, 197
Hypovolemic shocks, 323
Hypoxemia, 2, 16
Hysterectomy, 260

I

Ileus, 191
Impaction, 252
Increasing intracranial pressure, 142 - 143, 149
Infection, 101
Informed consent, 326

Inguinal hernia, 226
Insomnia, 376
Insulin, 161, 166
Intracellular fluid, 404
Intravascular coagulopathy, 268
Intravenous heparin, 114
Intravenous pyelogram, 231
Iron, 111
Iron dextram (Imferon), 112
Isometric exercises, 189
Isoniazid, 44

J

Jugular venous distentions, 67

K

Kaposi's sarcoma, 92, 95
Kernig's sign, 378
Ketoacidosis, 163
Kirschner wire, 207
Kussmaul, 50
Kussmaul breathing, 219

L

Laryngectomy, 363
Lasix, 84, 175, 359
Lead poisoning, 329
Left ventricular failure, 65 - 66
Leukemia, 117, 120 - 121
Level of consciousness, 2, 157
Levo-Thyroxine, 170 - 171
Levodopa, 155

M

Malignant hyperthermia, 332
Mantoux, 43
Mantoux test, 44

Marrow, 119, 414
Melanoma, 317
Ménière's syndrome, 290
Meningitis, 103
Mestinon, 152
Metabolic alkalosis, 349
Miotics, 288
Morphine, 3, 84
Morphine sulfate, 373 - 374
Musculoskeletal system, 187
Myasthenia gravis, 150
Mydriatics, 280, 282, 298
Myocardial infarction, 77 - 80

N

Narcan, 389
Nasogastric tube, 252 - 253
Negligence, 377
Nervous system, 133
Neurological assessment, 10
Neurovascular checks, 188, 193
Nitroglycerin, 61, 63
NPH, 168

O

Orthopnea, 64
Osteoarthritis, 200
Osteomyelitis, 204
Otitis media, 294
Oxygen, 56, 129, 198

P

Pain, 126, 188, 196, 204, 220, 269, 309, 316, 335, 407
Pancreatitis, 255
Paralysis, 146
Parkinson's disease, 154

Paroxysmal nocturnal dyspnea, 65, 70
Partial thromboplastin time (PPT), 113, 116
Patient-controlled analgesia (PCA), 341
PEEP, 3, 84
Pelvic traction, 209
Penicillin, 99, 411
Peptic ulcers, 236
Pericardial friction rub, 88
Pericarditis, 88
Peripheral edema, 14, 67, 70
Peripheral resistance, 74
Peripheral vascular disease, 382
Peritoneal dialysis, 231
Peritonitis, 410
Petechiae, 105, 113
Placebos, 342
Plaster cast, 188
Platelets, 395
Pneumocystis carinii, 22, 92
Pneumonia, 2, 22, 24
Pneumothorax, 26, 352
Point of maximal impulse, 89
Poisoning, 391
Polycythemia vera, 131
Portal hypertension, 76
Potassium, 357 - 358
Potassium depletion, 396
Potassium replacement, 371
Prostatitis, 269
Protamine sulfate, 369
Prothrombin time (PT), 113, 145, 398
Psoriasis, 400
Pulmonary edema, 64, 70, 83
Pulmonary embolism, 29, 115
Pulmonary embolus, 32

Pulse pressure, 74
Pyelonephritis, 212

R

Radiation, 9, 315
Range of motion, 193
Range of motion (ROM), 30
Regular insulin, 164
REM, 383
Renal calculi, 214
Renal failure, 217
    Diuretic phase, 217
    Recovery phase, 217
    Oliguric phase, 217
Renal function, 228
    Renal system, 211
Renal transplant, 230
Reproductive system
    Female, 259
    Male, 259
Respiratory acidosis, 34
Respiratory distress, 37
Respiratory emergency, 153
Respiratory isolation, 44
Restlessness, 26, 29, 31, 37, 83, 318
Restraints, 402
Rhonchi, 53
Ringer's lactate, 324

S

Schilling Test, 123 - 124
Septic shock, 348
Septicemia, 104
Serotonin, 384
Serum transaminase, 247
Shock, 115, 344

Sinusitis, 47
Sleep, 383 - 384, 386 - 387
Snellen chart, 300
Sodium, 357
Sputum specimen, 55
Steinmann's pin, 207
Stomatitis, 311
Strict isolation, 307
Stridor, 28, 37
Subarachnoid hemorrhage, 320
Subcutaneous emphysema, 365
Suctioning, 38, 40
Swan-Ganz catheter, 72
Syndrome of inappropriate ADH secretion , 174
Syphilis, 352
Systemic lupus erythemous (SLE), 105

T

Tachycardia, 110
Tagamet, 237 - 238, 392
Tension pneumothorax, 28
Tetanus toxid, 199
Tetany, 332, 402
Theophylline, 18
Thomas splint, 207
Thoracentesis, 364, 403, 405
Thrombus, 33
Tic douloureux, 394
TNM system, 308
Toxic shock syndrome (TSS), 266
Tracheostomy, 37, 40
Traction, 207
Transfusion reaction, 130
Transurethral prostatectomy (TURP), 276
Triage, 392

Tuberculosis, 43, 45, 92, 103
Tylenol, 203, 409

U

Universal precautions, 44, 95, 102, 104
Urinary calculi, 229
Urinary system, 211
Urinary tract infection, 212, 223
Urinary tract infection (UTI), 220
Urine, 224 - 225, 229
Urine specimen, 227

V

Ventricular fibrillation, 306
Vesicular, 53
Visual acuity, 284
Vital signs, 411
Vitamin B12, 123
Vitamin K, 321, 396

W

Walker, 202
Western blot test, 94
Wheezes, 49, 54
Wheezing, 38, 83

Skidmore-Roth Publishing, Inc. Order Form
1(800) 825-3150

Qty.	Title	Price	Total
	1994 Nurse's Trivia Calendar	$9.95	
	RN NCLEX Review Cards, 2nd Ed.	$24.95	
	PN/VN Review Cards	$24.95	
	Nurse's Survival Guide, 2nd Ed.	$24.95	
	The Body in Brief, 2nd Ed.	$26.95	
	The OSHA Handbook	$79.95	
	The OBRA Guidelines for Quality Improvement in Long Term Care	$59.95	
	Diagnostic & Laboratory Cards, 2nd Ed.	$23.95	
	Drug Comparison Handbook	$29.95	
Tax of 8.25% applies to Texas residents only. UPS ground shipping $5 for first item, $1 each additional item.		Subtotal	
		8.25% Tax	
		Shipping	
		TOTAL	

Name	
Company	
Address	
City	
State	Zip
Phone	

____ Check enclosed   ____ Visa   ____ MasterCard

Credit Card Number

Card Holder Name

Signature   Expiration Date

For fastest service call, 1-800-825-3150 or fax your order to us at (915) 877-4424. Orders are accepted by mail.

Skidmore-Roth Publishing, Inc.
7730 Trade Center Avenue • El Paso, TX • 79912